CHAIR YOGA FOR CAREGIVERS

Self-care Practices to Relieve Stress and Restore Balance

Copyright (c) 2024 **Jerome Woodworth**.

All rights reserved. No part of this publication may be reproduced, distributed, or transmitted in any form or by any means, including photocopying, recording, or other electronic or mechanical methods, without the prior written permission of the publisher, except in the case of brief quotations embodied in critical reviews and certain other non-commercial uses permitted by copyright law.

TABLE OF CONTENTS

Introduction

Caring for a loved one can be one of the most rewarding experiences in life, but it can also be incredibly challenging. As caregivers, we often find ourselves navigating a delicate balance between meeting the needs of our loved ones and taking care of ourselves. Yet, in the midst of our caregiving responsibilities, it's all too easy to overlook our own well-being.

But what if there was a way to find moments of peace, rejuvenation, and self-care amidst the demands of caregiving? What if there was a tool that could help us relieve stress, ease tension, and restore balance to our lives?

Now, let me introduce you to Sarah. She's been caring for her aging mother for the past five years, juggling her caregiving responsibilities alongside a demanding job and family commitments...

As much as Sarah loves her mother and finds fulfillment in caring for her, the constant stress and strain have taken a toll on her own well-being.

Like many caregivers, Sarah often finds herself neglecting her own needs in favor of prioritizing the needs of her loved one. She pushes through exhaustion, muscle tension, and emotional fatigue, believing that self-sacrifice is an inevitable part of caregiving.

But one day, Sarah discovers something that changes everything: chair yoga.

At first, Sarah was skeptical. How could simple yoga poses practiced from a chair possibly make a difference in her busy life? However, out of sheer desperation for relief, she decided to give it a try.

To her surprise, Sarah found that even a few minutes of chair yoga each day made a remarkable difference in how she felt. The gentle stretches eased the tension in her neck and shoulders, the deep breathing exercises calmed her racing mind, and the guided meditations provided moments of peace amidst the chaos.

Slowly but surely, Sarah began to carve out time for herself each day, practicing chair yoga as a form of self-care. As she continued her practice, she noticed profound changes not only in her physical well-being but also in her mental and emotional resilience.

Inspired by her own transformation, Sarah realized that chair yoga wasn't just a series of poses; it was a lifeline a way for caregivers like herself to find moments of solace, strength, and self-compassion in the midst of their caregiving journey.

And so, the idea for "Chair Yoga for Caregivers: Self-care Practices to Relieve Stress and Restore Balance" was born.

In this book, we'll explore the transformative power of chair yoga for caregivers, offering practical tools, gentle practices, and compassionate guidance to support you on your self-care journey. Whether you're in need of stress relief, physical rejuvenation, or simply a moment of peace, chair yoga has something to offer you. So, dear caregiver, take a deep breath, settle into your chair, and let's embark on this journey of self-care together. Because just like Sarah, you deserve to find moments of solace, strength, and serenity amidst the challenges of caregiving.

Understanding the Importance of Self-care for Caregivers

Caregiving is a deeply rewarding yet demanding role that often comes with significant physical, emotional, and mental strain. As caregivers, we devote ourselves to the well-being of our loved ones, often at the expense of our own health and happiness. However, neglecting our own needs can have profound consequences, not only for ourselves but also for those we care for.

Self-care is not selfish; it is an essential component of effective caregiving. Just as we cannot pour from an empty cup, we cannot effectively care for others if we neglect our own well-being. Understanding the importance of self-care is crucial for caregivers to maintain their health, resilience, and sense of fulfillment.

Physical Health: Caregiving can take a toll on our physical health, leading to exhaustion, muscle tension, and chronic conditions. Engaging in regular exercise, nutritious eating, and adequate rest are essential for caregivers to maintain their physical well-being. Chair yoga offers a gentle yet effective way to incorporate movement and relaxation into daily life, promoting flexibility, strength, and overall vitality.

Emotional Well-being: Caregiving is inherently emotional, often accompanied by feelings of stress, anxiety, and guilt. It's essential for caregivers to acknowledge and address their emotions, seeking support from friends, family, or professional counselors when needed. Chair yoga provides a safe space for caregivers to process their emotions, cultivate mindfulness, and find moments of peace amidst the chaos.

Mental Resilience: The demands of caregiving can be mentally taxing, leading to burnout and compassion fatigue. Cultivating mental resilience is vital for caregivers to navigate challenges with clarity and grace. Chair yoga offers techniques such as deep breathing, meditation, and visualization, which can help caregivers manage stress, enhance focus, and cultivate a positive mindset.

Relationships: Caregiving can strain relationships, leading to feelings of isolation and loneliness. Maintaining meaningful connections with friends, family, and support groups is essential for caregivers to feel supported and understood. Chair yoga provides an opportunity for caregivers to connect with others, whether through group classes or online communities, fostering a sense of belonging and camaraderie.

Quality of Care: Ultimately, self-care is not just about caregivers; it's about those we care for. When caregivers prioritize their well-being, they are better equipped to provide high-quality care to their loved ones. By investing in self-care practices like chair yoga, caregivers can enhance their energy, compassion, and resilience, creating a more nurturing and sustainable caregiving environment.

In essence, understanding the importance of self-care for caregivers is about recognizing our own inherent worth and value. By prioritizing our well-being, we honor ourselves and those we care for, fostering a culture of compassion, kindness, and resilience in the caregiving journey.

How Chair Yoga Can Benefit Caregivers

Being a caregiver is a demanding job that calls for mental clarity, emotional fortitude, and physical endurance. But in the thick of all the obligations and demands, caregivers often overlook their own health. Neglect like this can result in stress, burnout, and a general deterioration in health. Caregivers can greatly benefit from chair yoga's holistic approach to self-care in a number of ways.

Physical Well-being: Caregiving often involves long hours of sitting or standing, leading to muscle tension, stiffness, and fatigue. Chair yoga provides gentle stretches and movements that promote flexibility, improve circulation, and alleviate physical discomfort. Regular practice can help caregivers reduce muscle tension, increase range of motion, and enhance overall physical well-being.

Stress Reduction: Caregiving can be emotionally taxing, leading to feelings of stress, anxiety, and overwhelm. Chair yoga offers techniques such as deep breathing, mindfulness, and relaxation exercises that activate the body's relaxation response and reduce stress levels. By incorporating these practices into their daily routine, caregivers can find moments of calm amidst the chaos and cultivate greater resilience in the face of adversity.

Emotional Balance: The emotional demands of caregiving can take a toll on mental well-being, leading to mood swings, irritability, and emotional exhaustion. Chair yoga provides an opportunity for caregivers to tune into their emotions, release pent-up tension, and cultivate emotional balance. Through mindful movement and breath awareness, caregivers can enhance their emotional intelligence, cultivate self-compassion, and foster a greater sense of inner peace.

Mental Clarity: Caregiving requires constant multitasking, decision-making, and problem-solving, which can overwhelm the mind and lead to mental fatigue. Chair yoga offers practices that promote mental clarity, focus, and concentration. By incorporating mindful movement and breathwork into their routine, caregivers can clear mental clutter, enhance cognitive function, and improve mental acuity.

Self-care Ritual: Caregiving often leaves little time for self-care, as caregivers prioritize the needs of their loved ones above their own. Chair yoga offers a simple yet effective self-care ritual that caregivers can integrate into their daily routine. Whether it's a few minutes of deep breathing exercises or a gentle stretch break, chair yoga provides caregivers with an opportunity to prioritize their own well-being and nurture their body, mind, and spirit.

Community Connection: Caregiving can be isolating, as caregivers may feel disconnected from friends, family, and social activities. Chair yoga classes offer a supportive community where caregivers can connect with others who understand their experiences and share common challenges. By participating in group classes or online communities, caregivers can find solidarity, encouragement, and a sense of belonging.

In essence, chair yoga offers caregivers a holistic approach to self-care that addresses their physical, emotional, and mental well-being. By incorporating chair yoga into their daily routine, caregivers can cultivate resilience, reduce stress, and enhance their overall quality of life.

CHAPTER 1

The Caregiver's Journey

Overview of the Caregiver Experience

The caregiver's journey is a profound and multifaceted experience, characterized by a range of challenges, emotions, and responsibilities. Caregivers play a crucial role in providing physical, emotional, and often financial support to their loved ones who may be aging, ill, or disabled. This journey is not linear but rather a dynamic and evolving process that can vary greatly from one caregiver to another. Understanding the common experiences and challenges faced by caregivers is essential for providing effective support and resources.

Physical Demands: Caregiving often involves assisting with activities of daily living such as bathing, dressing, and feeding, which can be physically demanding. Caregivers may also need to manage medications, accompany their loved ones to medical appointments, and provide transportation. These physical tasks can take a toll on the caregiver's own health and well-being, leading to fatigue, muscle strain, and other physical ailments.

Emotional Rollercoaster: The emotional aspect of caregiving is perhaps one of the most challenging aspects to navigate. Caregivers may experience a wide range of emotions, including love, compassion, frustration, guilt, and grief. Witnessing the decline or suffering of a loved one can be emotionally exhausting, and caregivers may struggle to find a balance between their own needs and those of their loved ones.

Financial Strain: Providing care for a loved one can also have significant financial implications. Caregivers may need to reduce their working hours or leave their jobs altogether to provide full-time care. This loss of income can strain finances and impact long-term financial stability. Additionally, caregivers may incur expenses related to medical bills, home modifications, and other caregiving-related costs.

Social Isolation: Caregiving can be an isolating experience, particularly if caregivers are unable to maintain social connections outside of their caregiving role. Many caregivers report feeling lonely, disconnected, and unsupported, as their caregiving responsibilities may limit their ability to socialize or engage in leisure activities. This social isolation can exacerbate feelings of stress, depression, and burnout.

Role Strain: Balancing the responsibilities of caregiving with other roles and obligations can create significant strain for caregivers. Many caregivers juggle caregiving duties with work, parenting, household chores, and other responsibilities, leading to feelings of overwhelm and exhaustion. Finding time for self-care and personal fulfillment can be challenging amidst the demands of caregiving.

Despite these challenges, the caregiver's journey is also marked by moments of profound love, connection, and growth. Caregivers often develop deep bonds with their loved ones and find meaning and purpose in their caregiving role. By recognizing and validating the diverse experiences of caregivers, we can better support them in their journey and ensure they receive the resources and assistance they need to thrive.

Challenges Faced by Caregivers

Caregiving is an incredibly rewarding yet challenging journey, and I want to acknowledge the obstacles you may encounter along the way. As you dedicate yourself to the well-being of your loved ones, it's essential to recognize the challenges you may face and find ways to navigate them with resilience and support.

Physical Strain: You may find yourself grappling with the physical demands of caregiving, from assisting with mobility to managing household tasks. These responsibilities can take a toll on your body, leading to fatigue, muscle strain, and even injuries. It's crucial to prioritize your physical well-being and seek assistance when needed to prevent burnout.

Emotional Burden: The emotional aspects of caregiving can be overwhelming at times. You may experience a range of emotions, including stress, anxiety, grief, and guilt, as you witness the challenges your loved ones face. Remember to prioritize your mental health and seek support from friends, family, or counseling services when needed.

Financial Stress: Balancing caregiving responsibilities with financial obligations can be challenging. You may need to navigate reduced income, increased expenses, and complex insurance processes, all while providing the best possible care for your loved ones. Seeking financial assistance and exploring available resources can help alleviate some of this stress.

Social Isolation: Caregiving can be isolating, making it difficult to maintain social connections and relationships outside of your caregiving role. You may feel disconnected from friends, family, and community activities, leading to feelings of loneliness and isolation. Don't hesitate to reach out for support and stay connected with others who understand your experiences.

Role Strain: Balancing caregiving duties with other responsibilities, such as work, parenting, and household chores, can be overwhelming. You may struggle to find time for yourself and feel stretched thin between competing demands. Remember to prioritize self-care and set boundaries to avoid burnout.

Navigating the Healthcare System: Managing medical appointments, medications, and healthcare decisions can be complex and overwhelming. You may find yourself navigating unfamiliar medical terminology and procedures while advocating for your loved one's needs. Seeking guidance from healthcare professionals and support organizations can help you navigate this journey more effectively.

Guilt and Self-Care: It's common for caregivers to experience feelings of guilt when prioritizing their own needs and well-being. You may feel torn between caring for your loved ones and taking time for yourself, leading to feelings of guilt or neglect. Remember that self-care is not selfish; it's essential for maintaining your health and resilience as a caregiver.

Despite these challenges, your dedication, compassion, and resilience shine through in your caregiving journey. By acknowledging and addressing these challenges, you can better support yourself and your loved ones on this path.

The Importance of Self-care for Caregivers

Amidst the myriad responsibilities and challenges, you face in your caregiving role, it's crucial to recognize that your well-being matters just as much as the well-being of those you care for. Self-care isn't a luxury; it's a necessity for maintaining your physical, emotional, and mental health as you navigate the complexities of caregiving.

Prioritizing Your Health: As a caregiver, your health is paramount. Neglecting your own well-being can lead to burnout, exhaustion, and compromised health. By prioritizing self-care practices such as regular exercise, nutritious meals, and adequate rest, you can replenish your energy reserves and better cope with the demands of caregiving.

Managing Stress and Anxiety: Caregiving can be emotionally taxing, often leading to feelings of stress, anxiety, and overwhelm. Engaging in stress-reduction techniques such as meditation, deep breathing exercises, or mindfulness can help calm your mind and restore inner peace amidst the chaos.

Preventing Burnout: Caregiver burnout is a significant concern, characterized by physical, emotional, and mental exhaustion. Taking regular breaks, setting boundaries, and seeking respite care are essential strategies for preventing burnout and preserving your long-term well-being.

Nurturing Relationships: Maintaining connections with friends, family, and support networks is vital for your emotional health. Nurture your relationships, seek social support, and don't hesitate to lean on others when you need assistance or a listening ear.

Finding Joy and Fulfillment: While caregiving can be challenging, it also offers moments of profound joy and fulfillment. Take time to engage in activities that bring you happiness, whether it's pursuing hobbies, spending time in nature, or enjoying moments of quiet reflection.

Cultivating Resilience: Building resilience is essential for navigating the ups and downs of the caregiving journey. Embrace challenges as opportunities for growth, practice self-compassion, and celebrate your successes, no matter how small.

Seeking Support: You don't have to navigate the caregiving journey alone. Reach out for support from healthcare professionals, support groups, or counseling services. Sharing your experiences with others who understand can provide validation, encouragement, and valuable insights.

Remember, prioritizing self-care isn't selfish; it's an act of self-preservation and compassion. By caring for yourself, you're better equipped to care for those you love. Embrace self-care as an essential part of your caregiving journey, and know that you are worthy of the same care and compassion you so generously give to others.

CHAPTER 2
Chair Yoga Basics

Introduction to Chair Yoga

Welcome to the world of chair yoga, a gentle and accessible form of yoga that offers numerous benefits for individuals of all ages and abilities, including caregivers like yourself. In this chapter, we'll explore the fundamentals of chair yoga, its origins, and how it can be adapted to suit your unique needs and circumstances.

What is Chair Yoga? Chair yoga is a modified form of yoga that incorporates traditional yoga poses and practices while utilizing a chair for support and stability. Whether you're new to yoga or have physical limitations that make traditional yoga challenging, chair yoga offers a safe and effective way to experience the benefits of yoga practice.

Origins and Evolution: The roots of chair yoga can be traced back to the ancient traditions of yoga, where practitioners used props and supports to aid in their practice. Over time, chair yoga has evolved to become a recognized and respected form of yoga therapy, particularly beneficial for individuals with mobility issues, chronic pain, or other physical limitations.

Benefits of Chair Yoga: Chair yoga offers a wide range of benefits for caregivers and individuals alike. From improved flexibility and strength to reduced stress and enhanced relaxation, the gentle movements and mindful breathing techniques of chair yoga can support your overall well-being, both physically and mentally.

Accessible and Inclusive: One of the key advantages of chair yoga is its accessibility and inclusivity. Regardless of age, fitness level, or physical condition, chair yoga can be adapted to meet your unique needs and abilities. Whether you're recovering from an injury, managing a chronic condition, or simply looking for a gentle way to stay active, chair yoga offers a welcoming and supportive environment for all.

Getting Started: You don't need any special equipment or prior yoga experience to begin practicing chair yoga. All you need is a sturdy chair and a willingness to explore movement, breath, and mindfulness. Throughout this book, you'll discover a variety of chair yoga poses, sequences, and relaxation techniques designed to promote relaxation, reduce stress, and restore balance in your life.

Remember to approach every chair yoga practice with an open mind and a sense of curiosity as you begin your journey. Pay attention to your body, respect your boundaries, and acknowledge your accomplishments as you go. Your physical and mental well-being can be completely transformed by chair yoga, and you'll leave with the skills necessary to handle the difficulties of caregiving with fortitude and grace.

Benefits of Chair Yoga for Stress Relief and Balance Restoration

In the demanding role of caregiving, finding moments of peace and balance amidst the chaos is essential for your well-being. Chair yoga offers a gentle yet powerful means of relieving stress, restoring balance, and nurturing your overall health and vitality. In this section, we'll delve into the specific benefits of chair yoga for stress relief and balance restoration, empowering you to incorporate these practices into your daily life.

Stress Reduction: Caregiving often comes with its fair share of stressors, from managing medical appointments to handling unexpected challenges. Chair yoga provides a sanctuary of calm amidst the storm, offering gentle movements, breathwork, and relaxation techniques to soothe your nervous system and quiet your mind. By practicing chair yoga regularly, you can reduce the effects of stress on your body and mind, promoting greater resilience and emotional well-being.

Mind-Body Connection: Chair yoga invites you to cultivate a deeper connection between your body, mind, and breath. Through mindful movement and breath awareness, you can become more attuned to the present moment, fostering a sense of grounding and inner peace. By nurturing this mind-body connection, you can better cope with the demands of caregiving, responding to challenges with greater clarity, composure, and compassion.

Improved Flexibility and Mobility: Sitting for extended periods can lead to stiffness and discomfort in the body, exacerbating feelings of tension and stress. Chair yoga offers a gentle way to increase flexibility and mobility, with modified poses and gentle stretches designed to release tension in the muscles and joints. By incorporating regular chair yoga practice into your routine, you can improve your range of motion, reduce stiffness, and enhance your overall comfort and well-being.

Enhanced Balance and Stability: Caregiving often requires physical strength and stability, whether assisting with transfers or navigating uneven terrain. Chair yoga poses and balance exercises can help improve your balance and stability, strengthening the muscles that support you in your caregiving duties. By practicing these poses regularly, you can enhance your physical resilience, reduce the risk of falls, and move through your daily tasks with greater confidence and ease.

Emotional Resilience: Caregiving can evoke a wide range of emotions, from joy and fulfillment to frustration and exhaustion. Chair yoga provides a safe space to acknowledge and process these emotions, offering gentle movement and breathwork techniques to support emotional release and self-expression. By cultivating emotional resilience through chair yoga practice, you can navigate the ups and downs of caregiving with greater equanimity and grace.

Your physical, emotional, and mental health can all greatly benefit from including chair yoga into your everyday practice. Chair yoga provides a haven of self-care amidst the responsibilities of caregiving, whether you practice for a short while each day or set aside specific time for a longer practice. Accept these practices with open arms and a readiness to take care of yourself, understanding that taking care of your own health improves your capacity to take care of the people you love.

Getting Started with Chair Yoga: Tips and Precautions

It's crucial to approach your chair yoga practice with mindfulness, self-awareness, and a strong sense of compassion for yourself when you start off. Chair yoga is a gentle yet powerful approach to improve your health, but as with any physical activity, it's important to pay attention to your body's signals and put safety first. To assist you get started with chair yoga and get the most out of your practice, we'll go over some important pointers and safety measures in this section.

Choose a Sturdy Chair: Selecting the right chair is fundamental to your chair yoga practice. Opt for a sturdy chair with a flat seat and backrest, preferably without armrests, to allow for a full range of movement. Ensure that the chair is positioned on a stable surface, free from any hazards or obstacles that may impede your practice.

Listen to Your Body: One of the guiding principles of chair yoga is honoring your body's wisdom and limitations. As you move through each pose, pay close attention to how your body responds, and adjust the intensity or duration of the pose accordingly. If you experience discomfort or pain, gently come out of the pose and modify it to better suit your needs.

Practice Mindful Breathing: Breath awareness is a cornerstone of chair yoga practice, helping to calm the mind, reduce stress, and enhance the mind-body connection. Incorporate mindful breathing techniques into your practice, such as deep belly breathing or equal-length inhales and exhales, to promote relaxation and presence.

Modify Poses as Needed: Chair yoga offers a wide range of modified poses to accommodate varying levels of flexibility and mobility. Don't hesitate to modify poses to suit your individual needs, using props such as cushions or blocks for support and stability. Remember that there's no one-size-fits-all approach to yoga, and embracing modifications is an essential part of your practice.

Stay Hydrated: As you engage in chair yoga practice, remember to stay hydrated by drinking water before, during, and after your session. Hydration is key to supporting your body's functions and maintaining optimal health, especially during periods of physical activity.

Take Regular Breaks: While chair yoga offers gentle movement and relaxation, it's essential to listen to your body and take regular breaks as needed. If you feel fatigued or overwhelmed, pause your practice and take a moment to rest and rejuvenate. Remember that self-care is about honoring your body's needs and nurturing yourself with compassion and kindness.

Consult with Your Healthcare Provider: If you have any pre-existing medical conditions or concerns, it's advisable to consult with your healthcare provider before beginning a new exercise regimen, including chair yoga. Your healthcare provider can offer personalized guidance and recommendations based on your individual health status and medical history.

As you begin your chair yoga journey, keep in mind that your purpose is the most crucial component of your practice. With an open mind and a curious spirit, approach every session and embrace the transforming potential of chair yoga to nourish your body, mind, and soul.

CHAPTER 3

Chair Yoga Poses for Stress Relief

Gentle Neck and Shoulder Stretches

In our fast-paced lives, tension often accumulates in the neck and shoulders, manifesting as stiffness, discomfort, and even pain. As caregivers, these areas may bear the brunt of our responsibilities, holding onto stress and strain accumulated throughout the day. Fortunately, chair yoga offers a gentle yet effective way to release tension and restore mobility to these vital areas of the body.

Neck Rolls: Begin by sitting comfortably in your chair with your feet flat on the ground and your spine tall. Inhale deeply as you lengthen through the crown of your head, and exhale as you gently drop your right ear towards your right shoulder. Slowly roll your chin towards your chest, and then let your left ear drop towards your left shoulder. Continue this circular motion for several breaths, moving with awareness and ease. This gentle movement helps to release tension in the neck and increase flexibility.

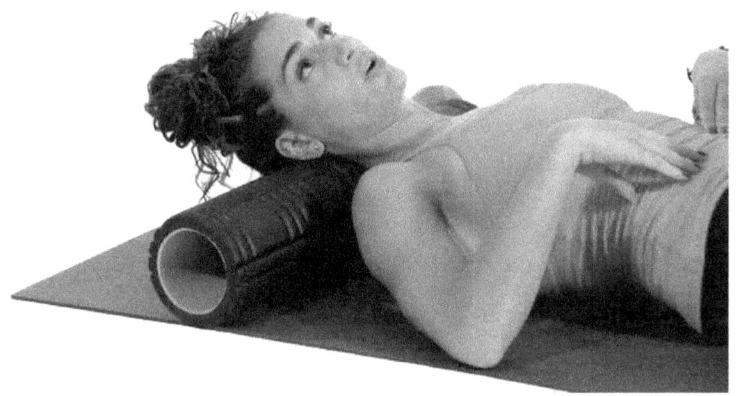

Shoulder Shrugs: Sit comfortably in your chair with your arms resting by your sides. Inhale deeply as you lift your shoulders towards your ears, squeezing them tightly towards each other. Exhale as you release your shoulders down and back, allowing them to relax and soften. Repeat this movement several times, synchronizing your breath with the movement of your shoulders. Shoulder shrugs are an excellent way to release built-up tension and promote circulation in the shoulder area.

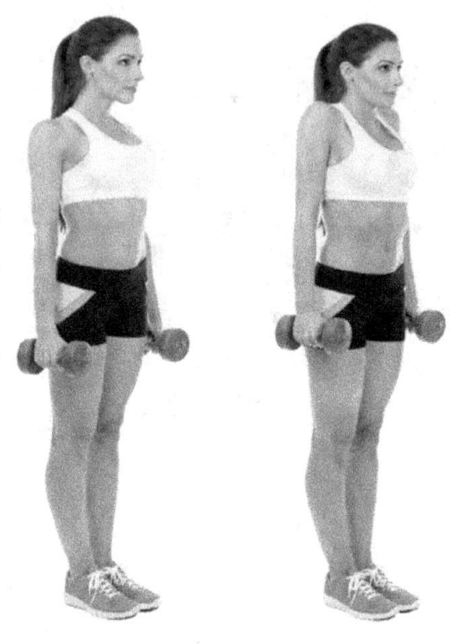

Eagle Arms: Sit tall in your chair and extend your arms out in front of you at shoulder height. Cross your right arm over your left arm, bringing your palms to touch if possible. If your palms don't touch, you can simply hold onto your shoulders with your hands. Lift your elbows slightly as you draw your shoulder blades down your back. Hold this pose for several breaths, feeling a deep stretch across your upper back and shoulders. Repeat on the other side by crossing your left arm over your right.

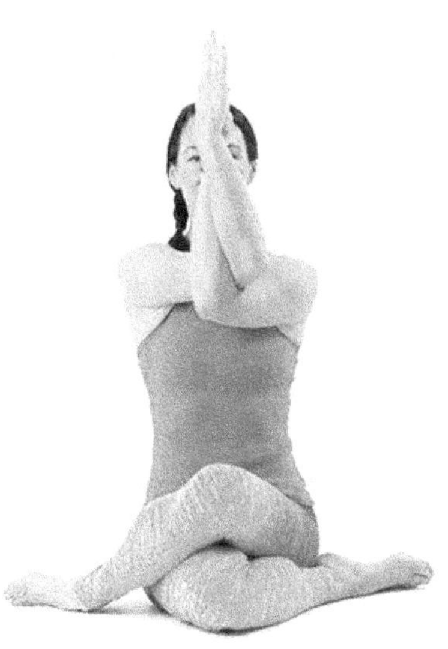

Seated Cat-Cow Stretch: Sit comfortably in your chair with your feet flat on the ground and your hands resting on your knees. Inhale deeply as you arch your spine, lifting your chest and gaze towards the ceiling. Exhale as you round your spine, tucking your chin towards your chest and drawing your belly button towards your spine. Continue flowing between these two movements with your breath, synchronizing each movement with an inhale or exhale. This gentle spinal movement helps to release tension in the neck, shoulders, and upper back while promoting flexibility and mobility.

Ear-to-Shoulder Stretch: Sit tall in your chair with your feet flat on the ground and your hands resting on your lap. Inhale deeply as you lengthen through the crown of your head, and exhale as you gently drop your right ear towards your right shoulder. Hold this stretch for several breaths, feeling a deep stretch along the left side of your neck and shoulder. Inhale to return to center, and then exhale as you repeat on the other side. This stretch helps to release tension in the neck and shoulders and can be particularly beneficial for relieving stiffness and discomfort.

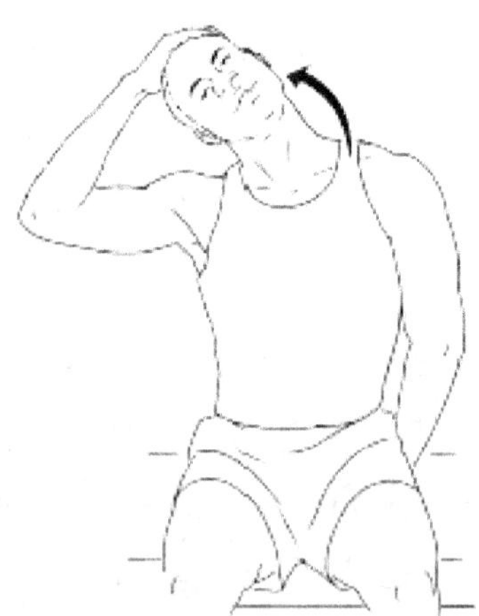

Thread the Needle Stretch: Sit tall in your chair with your feet flat on the ground and your hands resting on your knees. Inhale deeply as you reach your right arm up towards the ceiling, and exhale as you thread your right arm underneath your left arm, lowering your right shoulder towards the ground. Rest your right ear and cheek on the ground if possible, feeling a deep stretch across your upper back and shoulder. Hold this stretch for several breaths, allowing your body to relax and soften into the pose. Inhale to return to center, and then exhale as you repeat on the other side. This stretch helps to release tension in the shoulders, upper back, and neck, promoting relaxation and mobility.

These easy stretches for the neck and shoulders will help you release tension, ease discomfort, and bring balance back to these important body parts while you do chair yoga. As you explore each stretch, keep in mind to move consciously, breathe deeply, and pay attention to your body's signals. Regular practice can help you develop more ease, flexibility, and wellbeing in your shoulders and neck, which will improve your quality of life overall and help you in your position as a career.

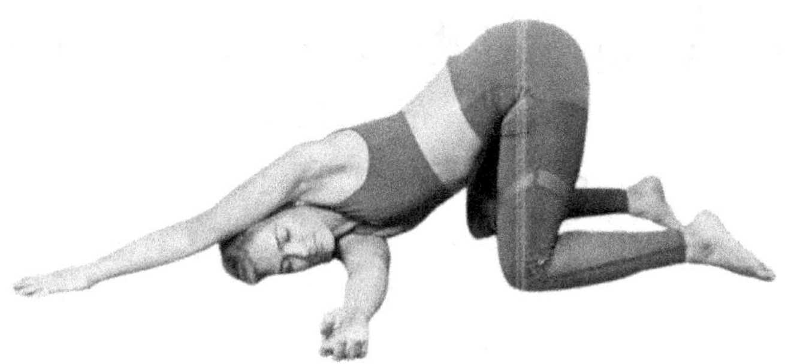

Seated Twists and Side Stretches

In the realm of chair yoga, seated twists and side stretches are gentle yet potent tools for relieving stress, improving flexibility, and rejuvenating both body and mind. These accessible poses target key areas of tension in the *spine, torso, and side body*, offering a welcome respite from the demands of caregiving and daily life. As you explore these movements, remember to move mindfully, honoring your body's unique needs and limitations, and allowing your breath to guide you deeper into each stretch.

Seated Twist: Begin by sitting tall in your chair, with your feet flat on the ground and your spine elongated. Inhale deeply, lengthening through the crown of your head, and exhale as you gently twist your torso to the right. Place your left hand on the outside of your right knee and your right hand on the back of the chair for support. With each inhale, lengthen your spine, and with each exhale, deepen the twist, gently wringing out tension from the spine. Hold the twist for several breaths, feeling the revitalizing effects of the stretch. Then, inhale to return to center and repeat on the other side. Remember to maintain a sense of ease and openness in the pose, avoiding any strain or discomfort.

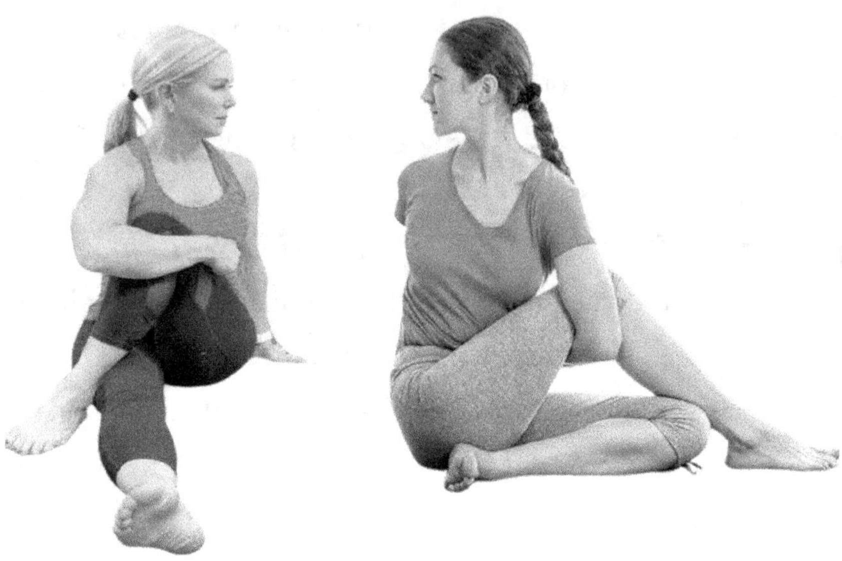

Side Stretch: Sit tall in your chair, grounding through both sit bones and lengthening through the spine. Inhale deeply, and as you exhale, reach your right arm overhead, leaning gently to the left side. Keep both feet firmly planted on the ground and both hips rooted in the chair. Feel the stretch along the right side of your body, from your fingertips down to your hip. Take several deep breaths in this position, allowing the breath to expand into the side body and create space and openness. Inhale to return to center, and then exhale as you repeat on the other side. With each stretch, cultivate a sense of surrender and relaxation, letting go of tension with each exhale.

Forward Fold with Side Stretch: From a seated position, inhale deeply, and as you exhale, hinge forward at the hips, folding your torso over your thighs. Allow your arms to hang loosely toward the floor, and if comfortable, reach your right hand toward your left foot or ankle. Inhale to lengthen through the spine, and as you exhale, deepen the stretch by leaning gently to the left side. Feel the lengthening and opening along the right side of your body, from the fingertips to the hip. Breathe deeply into this stretch, allowing the breath to soothe and nourish tight muscles and release tension. Inhale to return to center, and then exhale as you repeat on the other side. With each repetition, embrace the opportunity to find balance and harmony within the body and mind.

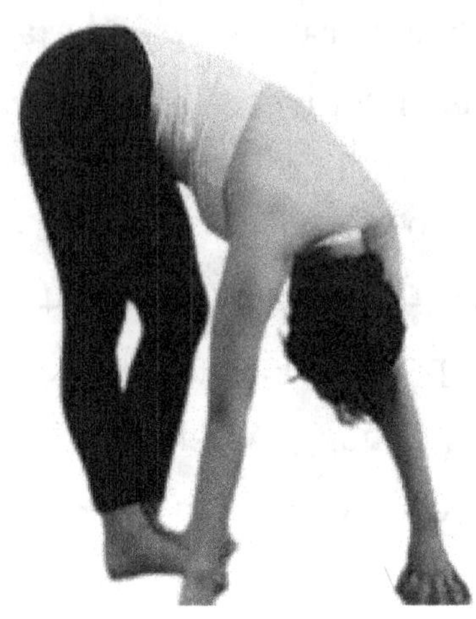

Tips for Practice: As you explore seated twists and side stretches, keep the following tips in mind to enhance your practice:

- Listen to your body and honor its wisdom. If you experience any pain or discomfort, ease out of the pose or modify as needed.

- Avoid overstretching: Stretch only to the point of mild discomfort, never to the point of pain.

- Focus on your breath, using each inhale to create space and each exhale to release tension.

- Move mindfully and with awareness, paying attention to the sensations in your body and the fluctuations of your mind.

- Experiment with variations and modifications to find what feels best for you in each pose.

Above all, approach your practice with kindness and compassion, nurturing yourself with each breath and movement.

By integrating seated twists and side stretches into your chair yoga practice, you can cultivate greater ease, flexibility, and relaxation in both body and mind. These gentle yet powerful movements offer a sanctuary of calm amidst the busyness of caregiving, supporting you in nurturing your well-being and restoring balance to your life.

Deep Breathing Exercises for Relaxation

Deep breathing techniques are potent anchors for relaxation in the chair yoga sanctuary, encouraging carers to establish a quiet inner voice among the stresses of life. These straightforward yet effective techniques provide a means to decompress, clear the mind, and revitalise the soul, promoting a profound sensation of calm and wellbeing. Allow your breath to lead you into a deep state of rejuvenation and relaxation as you set off on this voyage of introspection. **Diaphragmatic Breathing**: Begin by finding a comfortable seated position in your chair, placing your hands on your belly. Close your eyes, if comfortable, and take a deep breath in through your nose, allowing your abdomen to expand fully as you inhale. Feel the breath filling your belly, ribcage, and chest, and then exhale slowly through your mouth, allowing your belly to gently contract. Continue this pattern of deep, diaphragmatic breathing, focusing on the sensation of the breath moving in and out of your body. With each inhale, invite a sense of calm and ease to wash over you, and with each exhale, release any tension or stress held within. Allow yourself to sink deeper into relaxation with each breath, surrendering to the present moment and letting go of any worries or distractions.

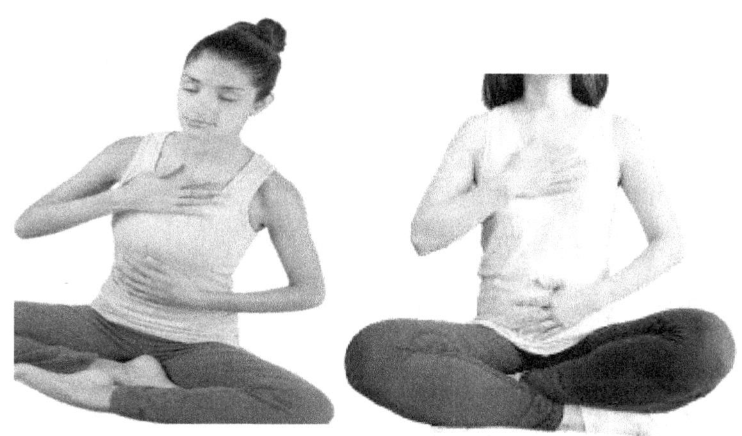

4-7-8 Breathing: Another effective technique for promoting relaxation is the 4-7-8 breathing exercise. Begin by inhaling deeply through your nose for a count of four seconds, feeling the breath fill your lungs completely. Hold your breath for a count of seven seconds, allowing the oxygen to saturate your cells and calm your nervous system. Then, exhale slowly and completely through your mouth for a count of eight seconds, releasing any tension or anxiety with each breath out. Repeat this cycle of breath for several rounds, allowing each inhale to nourish and rejuvenate you, and each exhale to cleanse and purify your body and mind. With each repetition of the 4-7-8 breathing exercise, feel yourself sinking deeper into a state of profound relaxation and serenity.

Alternate Nostril Breathing: This ancient yogic practice is known for its ability to balance the nervous system and calm the mind. Begin by sitting comfortably in your chair, with your spine tall and your shoulders relaxed. Close your right nostril with your right thumb and inhale deeply through your left nostril, counting to four as you breathe in. At the top of your inhale, close your left nostril with your ring finger, and release your thumb to exhale slowly through your right nostril, counting to eight as you breathe out. Then, inhale through your right nostril for a count of four, close both nostrils briefly at the top of your inhale, and exhale through your left nostril for a count of eight. Continue this pattern of alternating nostril breathing for several rounds, allowing each breath to calm and center you, and each exhale to release any tension or stress held within. Feel yourself becoming more grounded and centered with each breath, finding a sense of peace and equilibrium within.

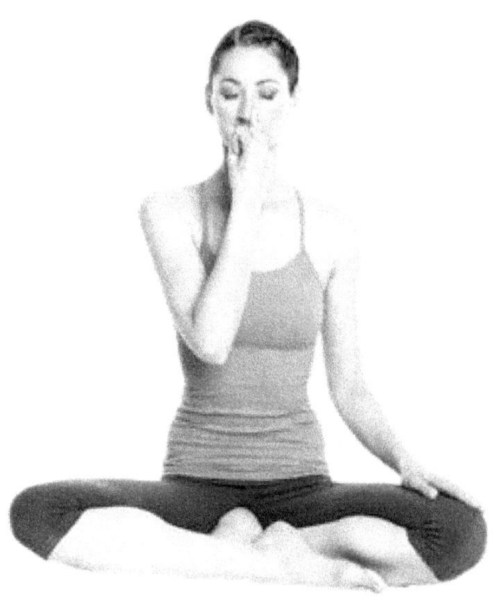

Tips for Practice: As you engage in deep breathing exercises for relaxation, keep the following tips in mind to enhance your experience.

- Find a quiet, comfortable space where you can practice without distractions.
- Set aside dedicated time each day for your breathing practice, even if it's just a few minutes.
- Experiment with different techniques to find what resonates most with you, and don't be afraid to modify as needed.

- Practice with gentle awareness and non-judgmental curiosity, allowing yourself to simply be with whatever arises.

Above all, acknowledge yourself and your individual self-care path by approaching your practice with kindness and compassion. You may create a haven of peace amid the chaos of caregiving by including deep breathing techniques into your chair yoga practice. This will nurture your well-being and help you regain equilibrium in your life. These straightforward yet effective techniques provide you with a path to inner calm and tranquillity and provide you the ability to face life's obstacles head-on and bounce back from them.

Guided Meditation and Mindfulness Practices

Guided meditation and mindfulness exercises are powerful tools for caregivers in the chair yoga sanctuary, providing an environment of calm and peace amidst the stresses of everyday life. With the help of these simple yet effective approaches, carers can develop present-moment awareness, lower stress levels, and promote a profound sense of inner peace and well-being. Allow the calming guidance of mindfulness and meditation to gradually lead you into a state of profound relaxation and refreshment as you set out on this journey of self-discovery and regeneration.

Body Scan Meditation: Begin by finding a comfortable seated position in your chair, with your feet flat on the floor and your hands resting on your thighs. Close your eyes, if comfortable, and take a few deep breaths to center yourself in the present moment. Begin to bring your awareness to different parts of your body, starting with your toes and gradually moving upward through your feet, ankles, calves, knees, and thighs. Notice any sensations, tensions, or areas of tightness as you scan each part of your body, and gently release any tension or discomfort with each exhale. Continue this process of scanning and releasing, moving slowly and mindfully through your entire body, until you reach the crown of your head. Allow yourself to sink deeper into relaxation with each breath, surrendering to the sensations of peace and tranquility that arise within.

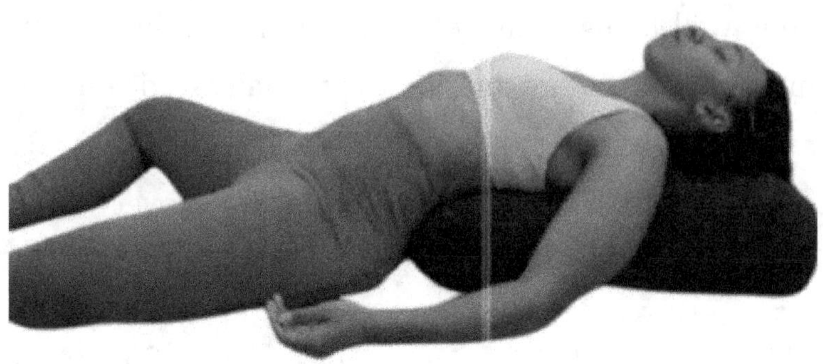

Breath Awareness Meditation: Another powerful practice for cultivating mindfulness is breath awareness meditation. Begin by finding a comfortable seated position in your chair, with your spine tall and your shoulders relaxed. Close your eyes, if comfortable, and bring your attention to your breath as it flows in and out of your body. Notice the sensation of the breath as it enters through your nostrils, fills your lungs, and expands your belly. Follow the natural rhythm of your breath, allowing it to guide you into a state of deep relaxation and presence. Whenever your mind begins to wander, gently bring your focus back to your breath, anchoring yourself in the present moment. With each inhale, invite a sense of calm and clarity to wash over you, and with each exhale, release any tension or stress held within. Allow yourself to simply be with your breath, surrendering to the ebb and flow of each inhale and exhale.

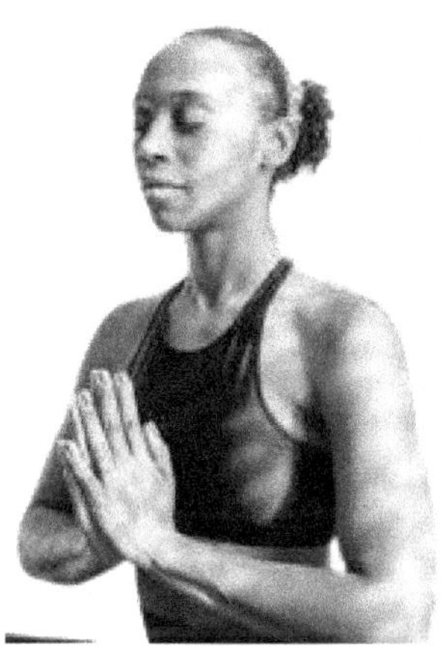

Loving-Kindness Meditation: This heart-centered practice is a beautiful way to cultivate compassion and connection towards yourself and others. Begin by finding a comfortable seated position in your chair, with your hands resting on your heart. Close your eyes, if comfortable, and take a few deep breaths to center yourself in the present moment. Begin to silently repeat the following phrases to yourself, allowing each word to resonate deeply within your heart: "May I be happy. May I be healthy. May I be safe. May I live with ease." Continue to repeat these phrases, extending feelings of love, kindness, and compassion towards yourself with each repetition. Once you feel a sense of warmth and tenderness towards yourself, gradually extend these wishes outward to others, starting with loved ones, friends, and caregivers, and then expanding to include all beings everywhere. Allow yourself to be enveloped in a sense of love and connection, knowing that you are held and supported by the infinite wellspring of compassion within.

Tips for Practice: As you engage in guided meditation and mindfulness practices, keep the following tips in mind to enhance your experience:

- Find a quiet, comfortable space where you can practice without distractions.
- Set aside dedicated time each day for your meditation practice, even if it's just a few minutes.
- Experiment with different techniques to find what resonates most with you, and don't be afraid to modify as needed.

- Approach your practice with gentle curiosity and non-judgmental awareness, allowing yourself to simply be with whatever arises.

Above all, be patient and compassionate with yourself, honoring your unique journey of self-discovery and self-care.

You may create a holy sanctuary of peace and tranquility amidst the chaos of caregiving by including mindfulness exercises and guided meditation into your chair yoga programme. This will nurture your well-being and help you regain balance in your life. These straightforward yet effective techniques provide a road to resilience and inner serenity, enabling you to face life's obstacles with poise and composure.

CHAPTER 4

Chair Yoga for Physical Well-being

Improving Posture and Alignment

As we transition into Chapter 4, "Chair Yoga for Physical Well-being," we embark on a journey to enhance posture and alignment through the transformative practice of chair yoga.

Imagine the hustle and bustle of daily life, where caregivers often find themselves caught in a whirlwind of responsibilities, their bodies contorted in uncomfortable positions as they tend to the needs of others. Now, envision the gentle embrace of chair yoga, offering a sanctuary of relief and restoration.

In the practice of chair yoga, finding better alignment and posture becomes a holy task. Caregivers are taken to a deep awareness of their bodies via intentional movements and mindful breathing, gently easing them back into balance and harmony.

At the heart of chair yoga lies the invitation to realign, to rediscover the natural grace and poise that reside within. With each posture, each gentle stretch, caregivers learn to release tension, to unfurl the knots of stress that have woven themselves into their muscles and joints.

Caregivers can recalibrate their bodies, realign their spines, and rediscover the innate power and resilience that reside within by using chair yoga as a retreat. It provides a brief break from the demands of caring for others, a breather in the middle of the mayhem.

Understanding that genuine well-being starts from within, we explore the nuances of posture and alignment as we go further into the practice of chair yoga. By engaging in these activities, carers nourish not only their bodies but also their spirits, finding comfort in the embrace of movement and awareness.

Strengthening Core Muscles

We explore the essential practice of strengthening core muscles in Chapter 4, "Chair Yoga for Physical Well-Being," to address the unique demands and difficulties experienced by care providers. Because their jobs frequently include lifting, bending, and extended durations of physical effort, carers must keep a strong and stable core in order to prevent accidents and to promote general well-being.

Core muscles, including those in the abdomen, lower back, hips, and pelvis, serve as the anchor for physical stability and resilience. By incorporating targeted chair yoga exercises, caregivers can effectively strengthen these muscles while addressing common issues such as poor posture, back pain, and fatigue.

One powerful exercise for strengthening the core is the Seated Spinal Twist. By gently rotating the torso while seated, caregivers engage the muscles along the spine and abdomen, promoting flexibility and stability. This exercise not only relieves tension in the back but also enhances spinal mobility, crucial for caregivers who may spend long hours in static positions.

Additionally, practicing Seated Pelvic Tilts and Kegel Contractions helps caregivers develop awareness and control over their pelvic floor muscles. Strengthening these muscles not only improves pelvic stability but also enhances bladder control, addressing a common concern among caregivers.

Through consistent practice of these chair yoga exercises, caregivers gradually experience a transformation in their physical well-being. They notice improvements in their posture, as their spine becomes more aligned and their shoulders relax. They also feel a renewed sense of energy and vitality, enabling them to meet the demands of caregiving with greater ease and resilience

Beyond the physical benefits, chair yoga offers caregivers a holistic approach to self-care, nurturing their mental and emotional well-being alongside their physical health. As caregivers prioritize their own self-care through these practices, they cultivate a sense of balance and inner peace, essential for navigating the challenges of caregiving with grace and compassion.

In essence, chair yoga for caregivers is not just about strengthening the body; it's about empowering caregivers to reclaim their vitality, resilience, and sense of well-being amidst the demands of their caregiving journey. Through mindful movement and breathwork, caregivers discover a sanctuary for self-nurturing and renewal, ensuring they have the strength and resilience to continue caring for others with love and compassion.

Enhancing Flexibility and Range of Motion

Caregivers are introduced to doable strategies for increasing range of motion and flexibility in Chapter 4, "Chair Yoga for Physical Well-Being," which is essential for reducing physical stress and increasing mobility.

Key Highlights:

Understanding the Need: Caregivers often experience muscle tightness and joint stiffness due to the demands of caregiving tasks, leading to discomfort and reduced mobility.

Accessible Practices: Chair yoga offers caregivers gentle yet effective exercises that are adaptable and suitable for all ages and fitness levels.

Targeted Movements: Specific chair yoga exercises focus on releasing tension, increasing flexibility, and improving range of motion in key areas of the body, such as the spine, hips, and shoulders.

Mind-Body Connection: By tuning into their breath and sensations, caregivers cultivate body awareness and mindfulness, facilitating greater ease of movement and relaxation.

Practical Steps and Approach:

Seated Forward Fold: Begin by sitting comfortably in a chair with feet flat on the floor. Inhale deeply, lengthening the spine, then exhale as you hinge forward from the hips, allowing the torso to fold over the thighs. Hold for a few breaths, feeling the stretch along the spine and backs of the legs. Repeat several times, gradually deepening the stretch with each exhale.

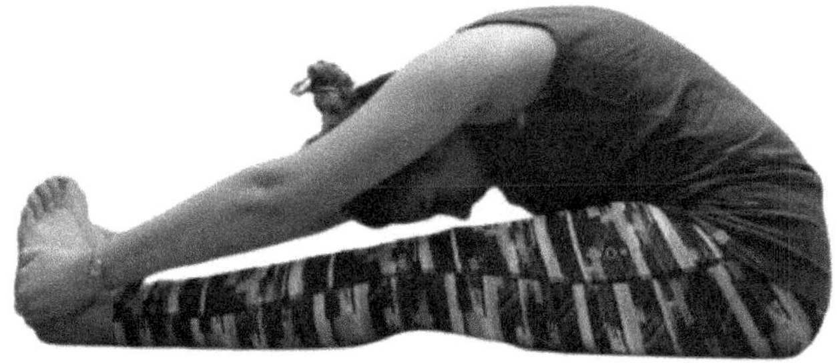

Seated Cat-Cow Stretch: While seated, place hands on knees. Inhale, arching the back and lifting the chest (Cow Pose). Exhale, rounding the spine and dropping the head forward (Cat Pose). Flow smoothly between these two positions, synchronizing movement with breath. Focus on elongating the spine and mobilizing each vertebra.

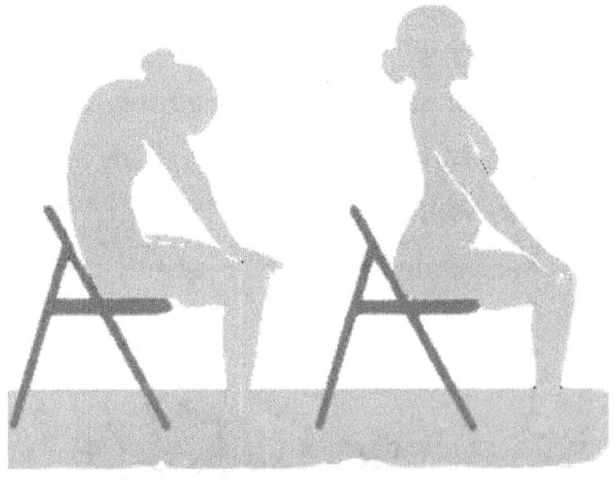

Seated Spinal Twist: Sit tall in the chair, placing the right hand on the backrest and the left hand on the right knee. Inhale to lengthen the spine, then exhale as you gently twist to the right, using the hands for support. Hold the twist for a few breaths, feeling the stretch along the spine. Repeat on the other side.

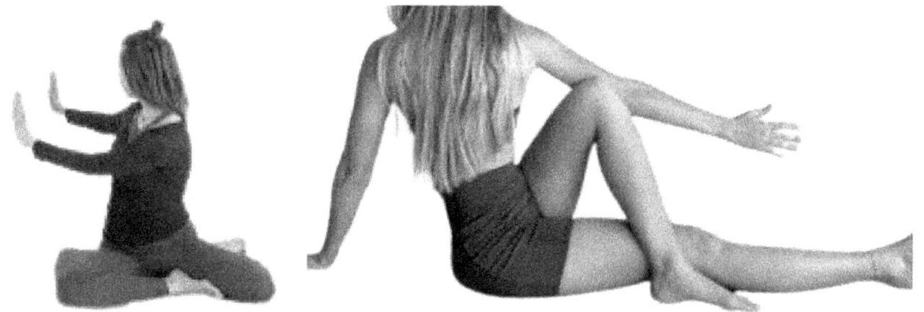

Seated Side Stretch: Sit with feet hip-width apart, arms extended overhead. Inhale deeply, then exhale as you lean to the right, stretching the left side of the body. Hold for a few breaths, feeling the lengthening sensation along the left side. Inhale back to center, then exhale to the other side.

Caregivers can see major gains in their flexibility, mobility, and general physical comfort by implementing these focused chair yoga techniques throughout their daily routine. Carers regain their vitality and well-being through regular practice and mindful awareness, which improves their capacity to care for their loved ones compassionately while also promoting their own health.

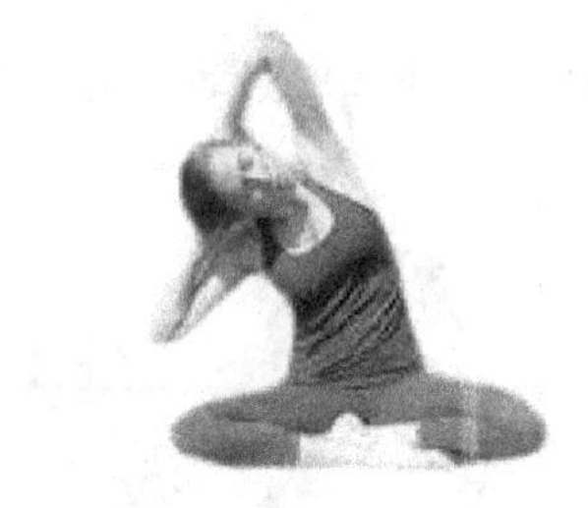

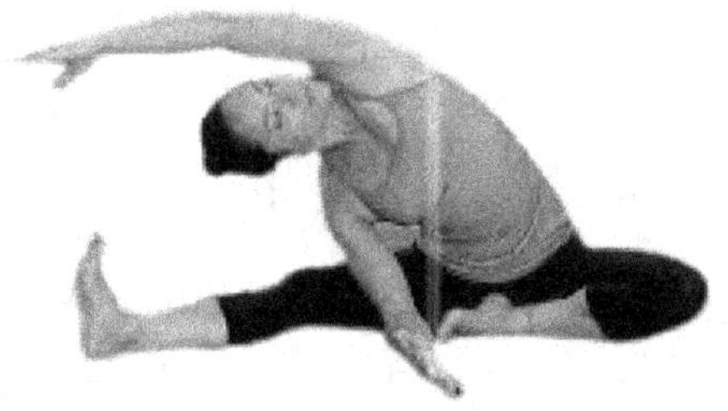

CHAPTER 5
Chair Yoga for Mental Well-being

Cultivating Emotional Resilience

Welcome, Caregivers, to the Chair Yoga Haven, a nurturing space crafted especially for you amidst the whirlwind of your daily responsibilities. Here, within the gentle folds of chair yoga, you'll discover a refuge where you can replenish your energy and restore your inner balance.

Amidst the tranquility of our haven, you'll be guided through gentle chair yoga practices meticulously designed to ease the burdens of your caregiving journey. With each mindful movement and deep breath, you'll embark on a voyage of self-care, nurturing your body, mind, and spirit along the way.

Within these comforting walls, you'll learn to cultivate emotional resilience, finding strength in vulnerability and grace in adversity. Mindfulness becomes your companion, anchoring you in the present moment and offering solace amidst life's challenges.

As you engage in chair yoga, you'll witness profound shifts within yourself. Tensions dissolve, muscles relax, and clarity emerges in your mind. With each practice, you reclaim ownership of your well-being, empowering yourself to navigate your caregiving role with renewed vigor and poise.

At the Chair Yoga Haven, you're not just participants; you're cherished guests on a sacred journey of self-nurturance and renewal. Here, you'll find respite from the demands of your caregiving duties, replenishing your spirit and rediscovering the joy and vitality within.

Step into the Chair Yoga Haven, carers, and discover the healing potential of self-care. Accept the gift of silence and recover your innate fortitude that reside within you.

Managing Anxiety and Depression

Caregiving can often lead to overwhelming feelings of anxiety and depression. As a caregiver, it's crucial to prioritize your mental well-being. Chair yoga offers effective techniques to manage these challenges and cultivate emotional resilience.

Breathwork for Calmness: Practice deep breathing exercises to calm the mind and reduce anxiety. Sit comfortably in your chair, close your eyes, and take slow, deep breaths. Focus on the sensation of your breath filling your lungs and exhale slowly. Repeat this process for a few minutes to alleviate stress and promote relaxation.

Mindful Movement: Engage in gentle chair yoga movements to promote mindfulness and alleviate depressive symptoms. Start with simple stretches and movements, paying close attention to the sensations in your body. Focus on the present moment, letting go of worries about the past or future. Mindful movement can help you feel more grounded and centered.

Positive Affirmations: Incorporate positive affirmations into your chair yoga practice to shift negative thought patterns and boost self-esteem. Repeat affirmations such as "I am capable and resilient" or "I am deserving of self-care and compassion." Affirmations can help reframe your mindset and cultivate a more positive outlook on life.

Guided Relaxation: Utilize guided relaxation techniques to release tension and promote emotional well-being. Close your eyes and visualize yourself in a peaceful and serene environment. Focus on relaxing each part of your body, starting from your toes and working your way up to your head. Allow yourself to let go of stress and tension with each exhale.

Journaling for Reflection: Take time to journal about your thoughts and emotions to gain insight into your mental well-being. Write freely about your experiences as a caregiver, expressing any feelings of anxiety or depression you may be experiencing. Journaling can provide a cathartic release and help you gain perspective on your emotions.

As a caregiver, you can effectively manage anxiety and despair by implementing these chair yoga practices into your daily routine. Never forget to put self-care first and ask for help when you need it to keep your mental health in check.

Enhancing Cognitive Function and Clarity

As a caregiver, maintaining mental clarity and cognitive function is essential for managing daily responsibilities effectively. Chair yoga offers invaluable techniques to sharpen your mind and enhance cognitive function.

Focused Breathing Exercises: Begin your chair yoga practice with focused breathing exercises to increase oxygen flow to the brain and improve concentration. Sit comfortably in your chair, close your eyes, and take slow, deep breaths. As you inhale, visualize oxygenated blood reaching your brain, revitalizing your mental faculties. Exhale slowly, releasing any tension or mental clutter. Repeat this process for several minutes to clear your mind and enhance focus.

Mindfulness Meditation: Incorporate mindfulness meditation techniques to cultivate mental clarity and present-moment awareness. Find a quiet space, sit comfortably in your chair, and close your eyes. Focus your attention on the sensations of your breath as it enters and exits your body. Notice any thoughts or distractions that arise without judgment, gently guiding your focus back to your breath. Mindfulness meditation can help reduce mental chatter and improve cognitive function over time.

Brain-Boosting Chair Yoga Poses: Engage in chair yoga poses specifically designed to stimulate brain activity and enhance cognitive function. Incorporate movements that involve crossing the midline of the body, such as alternating knee lifts or arm swings. These movements promote communication between the brain's hemispheres, improving coordination and cognitive processing. Additionally, practice seated spinal twists to stimulate blood flow to the brain and invigorate mental clarity.

Memory-Boosting Visualization: Utilize visualization techniques to improve memory retention and mental clarity. Close your eyes and visualize a place or scenario that brings you peace and tranquility. Engage your senses by imagining the sights, sounds, and smells of this imagined environment. Visualization exercises stimulate neural pathways associated with memory and cognition, enhancing mental clarity and recall.

Lifestyle Factors for Brain Health: In addition to chair yoga practices, prioritize lifestyle factors that support brain health and cognitive function. Maintain a balanced diet rich in brain-boosting nutrients such as omega-3 fatty acids, antioxidants, and vitamins. Stay physically active through regular exercise to promote blood flow to the brain and neuroplasticity. Adequate sleep, stress management, and social engagement are also essential for optimal cognitive function.

As a caregiver, you can support overall brain health, improve mental clarity, and improve cognitive function by implementing these chair yoga methods and lifestyle habits into your daily routine.

CHAPTER 6

Chair Yoga for Restorative Sleep

Relaxation Techniques for Better Sleep

As a caregiver, achieving restorative sleep is crucial for maintaining overall well-being and managing the demands of your role effectively. Chair yoga offers gentle relaxation techniques to promote deep, restful sleep and enhance your quality of life.

Progressive Muscle Relaxation: Begin your bedtime routine with progressive muscle relaxation to release tension and prepare your body for sleep. Find a comfortable seated position in your chair and close your eyes. Starting with your toes, progressively tense and then relax each muscle group in your body, working your way up to your head. Focus on the sensations of relaxation as tension melts away, promoting a sense of calm and tranquility conducive to sleep.

Guided Visualization: Incorporate guided visualization exercises to quiet the mind and create a peaceful mental landscape for sleep. Close your eyes and imagine yourself in a serene and tranquil setting, such as a peaceful beach or lush forest. Engage your senses by visualizing the sights, sounds, and sensations of this imagined environment. Allow yourself to become fully immersed in the experience, letting go of any worries or stressors that may be keeping you awake.

Deep Breathing Techniques: Practice deep breathing techniques to promote relaxation and activate the body's natural relaxation response. Sit comfortably in your chair with your feet flat on the ground and your hands resting on your lap. Inhale deeply through your nose, allowing your abdomen to expand fully. Exhale slowly through your mouth, letting go of any tension or stress with each breath. Repeat this deep breathing pattern for several minutes, focusing on the rhythm of your breath to quiet the mind and induce a state of relaxation.

Mindful Body Scan: Perform a mindful body scan to cultivate awareness of physical sensations and promote relaxation throughout your body. Close your eyes and bring your attention to your feet, noticing any sensations of warmth, tingling, or tension. Slowly move your awareness up through your body, paying attention to each area in turn, from your feet to the top of your head. With each breath, consciously release any tension or discomfort you may be holding onto, allowing yourself to sink deeper into a state of relaxation.

Soothing Soundscape: Create a soothing soundscape to promote relaxation and mask any disruptive noises that may interfere with sleep. Play soft, calming music or nature sounds such as gentle rainfall or ocean waves. Alternatively, use a white noise machine or smartphone app to generate a consistent, soothing sound that helps lull you into a deep and restful sleep.

To improve your general wellbeing as a caregiver and to encourage better sleep, incorporate these relaxing techniques into your nighttime routine. You may revitalise your body and mind by emphasising restful sleep, which will give you the resilience and energy you need to handle the responsibilities of caregiving with grace and vibrancy.

Bedtime Yoga Poses for Deep Rest

Prepare your body and mind for a restful night's sleep with these soothing bedtime yoga poses. Each pose is designed to release tension, calm the nervous system, and promote relaxation, helping you drift off into deep, restorative slumber.

Seated Forward Bend (Paschimottanasana): Begin by sitting comfortably in your chair with your feet flat on the ground and your spine tall. As you inhale, lengthen your spine, and as you exhale, gently hinge forward from your hips, allowing your torso to fold over your thighs. Relax your neck and shoulders, and let your head hang heavy. Hold the pose for a few breaths, feeling a gentle stretch in your lower back and hamstrings.

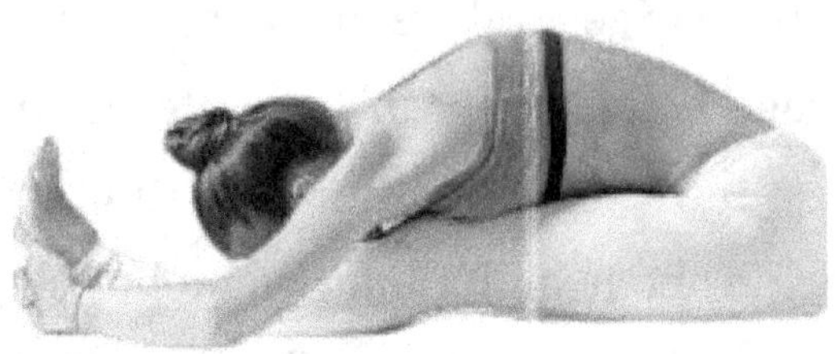

Seated Cat-Cow Stretch: Sit with your hands resting on your knees and your spine tall. Inhale as you arch your back and lift your chest towards the ceiling, drawing your shoulder blades together (cow pose). Exhale as you round your spine, tuck your chin to your chest, and draw your belly button towards your spine (cat pose). Flow between these two positions, moving with your breath, to release tension in your spine and promote relaxation.

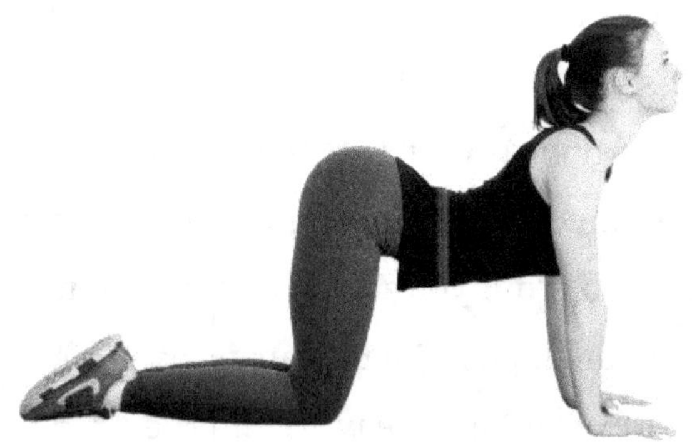

Seated Spinal Twist (Ardha Matsyendrasana):
Sit tall in your chair and place your right hand on the back of the chair. Inhale to lengthen your spine, then exhale to twist gently to the right, placing your left hand on the outside of your right thigh. Gaze over your right shoulder and take slow, deep breaths as you feel the twist in your spine. Hold for a few breaths, then repeat on the other side.

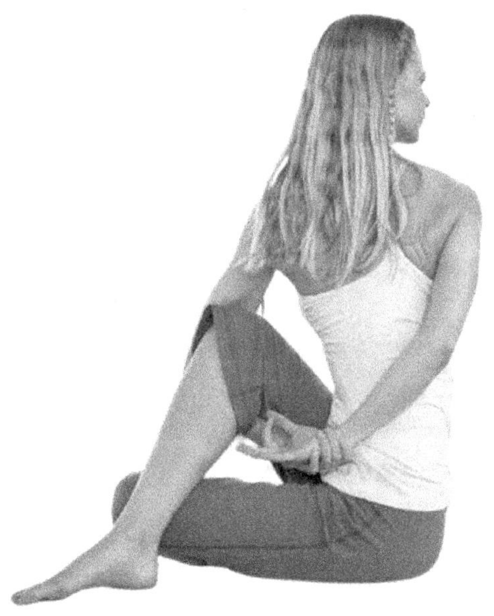

Legs-Up-The-Chair Pose (Viparita Karani): Sit close to a wall with your hips touching it. Extend your legs up the wall, resting them against it with your heels pointing towards the ceiling. Support your lower back by placing a folded blanket or cushion under your hips if needed. Close your eyes and relax into the pose, allowing the gentle inversion to promote relaxation and improve circulation.

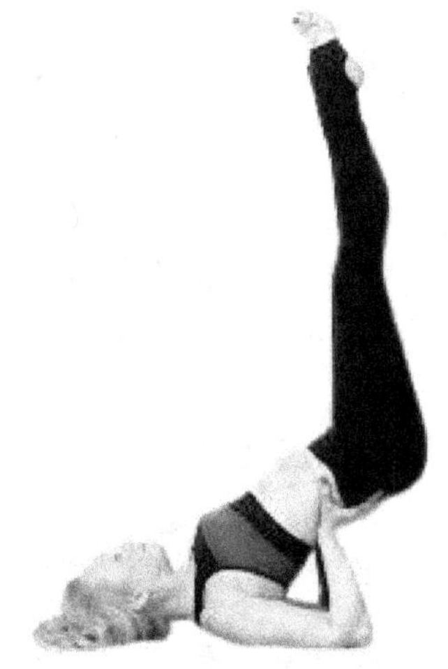

Supported Reclining Bound Angle Pose (Supta Baddha Konasana): Sit comfortably in your chair with your feet flat on the ground. Place a bolster or cushion behind you horizontally and lie back on it, allowing your spine to be fully supported. Bring the soles of your feet together and let your knees fall open to the sides. Rest your arms by your sides with your palms facing up. Close your eyes, breathe deeply, and allow yourself to surrender to the pose, releasing tension in your hips and groin.

Include these yoga positions for bedtime into your evening routine to help you decompress from the day and get ready for a restful sleep.

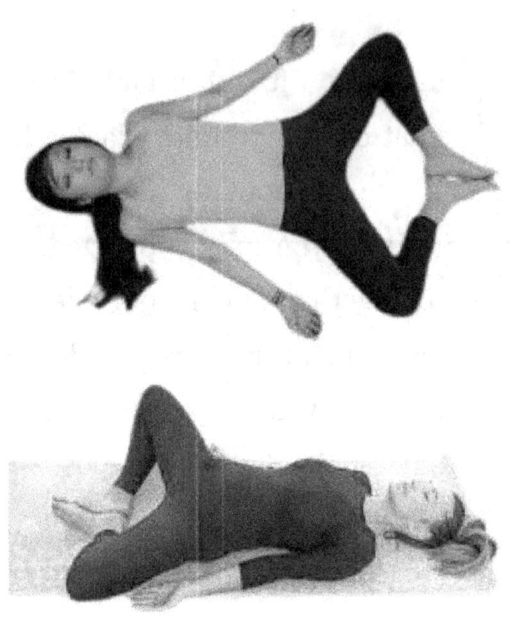

Creating a Relaxing Sleep Environment

Your sleep environment plays a crucial role in the quality of your restorative sleep. By setting up a relaxing atmosphere conducive to sleep, you can enhance your ability to unwind, fall asleep faster, and enjoy a deeper, more restful slumber. *Here are some tips for creating a sleep sanctuary:*

Dim the Lights: Lowering the lights in your bedroom signals to your body that it's time to wind down and prepare for sleep. Consider using dimmer switches or installing soft, ambient lighting to create a calming atmosphere.

Declutter Your Space: A clutter-free bedroom promotes relaxation and reduces stress. Take a few minutes each day to tidy up your space, clearing away any clutter or unnecessary items that may distract you from sleep.

Choose Comfortable Bedding: Invest in high-quality, comfortable bedding that promotes relaxation and supports restful sleep. Opt for soft, breathable fabrics and choose a mattress and pillows that provide adequate support for your body.

Create a Relaxing Bedtime Routine: Establishing a consistent bedtime routine can signal to your body that it's time to unwind and prepare for sleep. Incorporate relaxing activities such as reading, gentle stretching, or practicing meditation or deep breathing exercises to help calm your mind and body before bed.

Limit Electronic Devices: The blue light emitted by electronic devices can interfere with your body's natural sleep-wake cycle, making it harder to fall asleep. Limit screen time before bed and consider implementing a "digital curfew" to give your brain time to relax and prepare for sleep.

Use Relaxation Techniques: Incorporate relaxation techniques such as guided imagery, progressive muscle relaxation, or aromatherapy into your bedtime routine to help calm your mind and promote relaxation. Experiment with different techniques to find what works best for you.

Create a Peaceful Atmosphere: Enhance your sleep environment with soothing sounds or white noise to drown out any disruptive noises that may disturb your sleep. Consider using a white noise machine, calming music, or nature sounds to create a peaceful atmosphere conducive to sleep.

By creating a relaxing sleep environment, you can optimize your sleep quality and enjoy the benefits of deep, restorative rest. Experiment with these tips to find what works best for you and make adjustments as needed to create your ideal sleep sanctuary.

CHAPTER 7

Chair Yoga for Mindful Caregiving

Practicing Presence and Compassion

As a caregiver, cultivating presence and compassion is essential for providing attentive and empathetic care to your loved one. Chair yoga offers valuable tools and practices to support you in this endeavor, helping you stay grounded, centered, and compassionate in the face of caregiving challenges. Here's how you can incorporate presence and compassion into your caregiving journey through chair yoga:

Mindful Breathing: Begin by tuning into your breath, using it as an anchor to the present moment. Practice deep, intentional breathing exercises to calm your nervous system and cultivate a sense of inner peace and presence. With each breath, invite a sense of compassion and kindness towards yourself and your loved one.

Body Awareness: Through gentle chair yoga poses and movements, cultivate awareness of your body and its sensations. Pay attention to areas of tension or discomfort, and use mindful movement and gentle stretches to release tension and promote relaxation. As you move, maintain a sense of compassion towards your body, honoring its needs and limitations.

Compassionate Listening: Practice active listening with an open heart and mind, offering your full presence and attention to your loved one. Create a safe and supportive space for them to express themselves without judgment or interruption. Validate their feelings and experiences with empathy and compassion, fostering a deep sense of connection and understanding.

Self-Compassion: Remember to extend compassion and kindness towards yourself as well. Recognize the challenges and difficulties of caregiving, and offer yourself the same level of care and compassion that you provide to others. Practice self-care through chair yoga, meditation, or other nurturing activities that replenish your energy and restore your sense of well-being.

Cultivating Gratitude: Cultivate gratitude for the opportunity to serve as a caregiver and make a positive impact in your loved one's life. Take moments throughout the day to reflect on the blessings and joys that caregiving brings, even amidst the challenges. Cultivating a grateful heart can shift your perspective and help you find meaning and fulfilment in your caregiving role.

You may nurture your own resilience and well-being as a carer while improving the quality of care you give to your loved one by engaging in chair yoga practices that emphasise presence and compassion. Recognise that the people you look after benefit much from your presence and compassion, so embrace these practices with an open heart and a spirit of goodwill.

Setting Boundaries and Prioritizing Self-care

As a caregiver, it's natural to devote yourself wholeheartedly to the well-being of your loved one. However, it's equally important to establish healthy boundaries and prioritize your own self-care to prevent burnout and maintain your overall well-being. Chair yoga offers invaluable practices to help you set boundaries and prioritize self-care amidst your caregiving responsibilities. Here's how you can integrate these practices into your daily routine:

Self-Reflection: Begin by taking time for self-reflection to identify your personal needs, limits, and boundaries. Reflect on your caregiving role and the areas where you may be experiencing overwhelm or exhaustion. Recognize that setting boundaries is not selfish but essential for preserving your mental, emotional, and physical health.

Clear Communication: Communicate openly and assertively with your loved one and other family members about your caregiving boundaries and needs. Clearly articulate your limitations, availability, and the support you require to fulfill your caregiving responsibilities effectively. Setting clear boundaries fosters mutual understanding and respect within your caregiving dynamic.

Self-care Practices: Incorporate regular self-care practices into your daily routine to replenish your energy and prevent caregiver burnout. Dedicate time each day to engage in activities that nourish your mind, body, and spirit, such as chair yoga, meditation, journaling, or spending time in nature. Prioritize activities that bring you joy, relaxation, and fulfillment.

Chair Yoga for Boundaries: Practice chair yoga poses and mindfulness exercises that promote a sense of inner strength, resilience, and boundary-setting. Engage in grounding poses, such as Mountain Pose or Warrior Pose, to cultivate a strong and stable foundation within yourself. Use breathing techniques, such as Alternate Nostril Breathing, to calm the mind and center yourself amidst challenging situations.

Seeking Support: Don't hesitate to seek support from friends, family members, or professional caregivers when needed. Reach out to local support groups or online communities for caregivers to connect with others who understand your experiences and offer guidance and encouragement. Remember that asking for help is a sign of strength, not weakness.

Mindful Time Management: Practice mindful time management techniques to allocate your time and energy effectively between caregiving duties and self-care activities. Prioritize tasks based on their importance and urgency, and delegate responsibilities whenever possible. Set realistic expectations for yourself and avoid overcommitting to avoid unnecessary stress and overwhelm.

By setting boundaries and prioritizing self-care through chair yoga and mindful caregiving practices, you can cultivate a healthy balance between meeting your loved one's needs and honoring your own well-being. Embrace these practices with compassion and self-compassion, knowing that you deserve to be cared for just as much as you care for others.

Cultivating Gratitude and Acceptance

In the midst of the challenges and demands of caregiving, cultivating gratitude and acceptance can serve as powerful antidotes to stress and foster a greater sense of peace and contentment. Chair yoga offers practical tools and mindfulness practices to help caregivers cultivate gratitude for the present moment and accept the realities of their caregiving journey. Here's how you can integrate these practices into your daily life:

Gratitude Journaling: Dedicate time each day to reflect on the things you are grateful for in your caregiving experience. Keep a gratitude journal and write down three things you are thankful for, whether it's a supportive friend, a moment of joy with your loved one, or a simple act of kindness from a stranger. Focusing on gratitude can shift your perspective and bring attention to the positive aspects of your caregiving role.

Mindful Awareness: Practice mindful awareness of the present moment, accepting each moment as it unfolds without judgment or resistance. Use chair yoga and mindfulness techniques to anchor yourself in the here and now, letting go of worries about the past or future. Embrace each moment with openness and curiosity, noticing the beauty and blessings that surround you even amidst the challenges of caregiving.

Compassionate Self-talk: Cultivate self-compassion and kindness towards yourself as you navigate the ups and downs of caregiving. Offer yourself words of encouragement and support, acknowledging the efforts you are making and the love you are giving to your loved one. Treat yourself with the same level of care and compassion that you would extend to a dear friend facing similar challenges.

Gratitude Rituals: Create simple gratitude rituals to infuse your daily life with moments of appreciation and reflection. Start or end each day with a gratitude practice, such as lighting a candle and expressing thanks for the blessings in your life, or taking a mindful walk outdoors and noticing the beauty of nature. Find small ways to incorporate gratitude into your daily routine to uplift your spirits and foster a sense of abundance.

Chair Yoga for Acceptance: Use chair yoga poses and gentle movements to cultivate acceptance of your caregiving journey and the emotions that arise along the way. Practice poses that promote surrender and release, such as Child's Pose or Forward Fold, allowing yourself to let go of tension and resistance. Embrace the ebb and flow of caregiving with grace and equanimity, knowing that each moment is an opportunity for growth and learning.

Connection and Support: Seek connection and support from others who understand the challenges of caregiving and can offer empathy and validation. Join a caregiver support group, attend a chair yoga class for caregivers, or participate in online forums where you can share your experiences and receive encouragement from fellow caregivers. Remember that you are not alone on this journey, and there is strength in seeking support and solidarity.

By cultivating gratitude and acceptance through chair yoga and mindful caregiving practices, you can find greater peace, resilience, and joy in your caregiving journey. Embrace each moment with an open heart and a spirit of gratitude, knowing that you have the inner resources and support to navigate whatever challenges may arise.

CHAPTER 8

Chair Yoga for Connection and Community

Partner and Group Chair Yoga Practices

Chair yoga offers a wonderful opportunity for caregivers to connect and bond with their loved ones or fellow caregivers through partner and group practices. These interactive sessions not only promote physical well-being but also foster a sense of connection, support, and community. Here are some partner and group chair yoga practices to explore:

Partner Chair Yoga Poses: Invite a loved one or caregiver to join you in a series of partner chair yoga poses. Sit facing each other on chairs, holding hands or gently touching palms. Explore synchronized movements such as gentle twists, side stretches, and shoulder rolls, mirroring each other's actions and breathing in harmony. Partner chair yoga can deepen your connection with your partner or caregiver while promoting relaxation and joint mobility.

Chair Yoga Circles: Gather a group of caregivers or friends in a circle of chairs for a chair yoga session. Begin with a brief centering meditation or breathing exercise to cultivate a sense of presence and connection. Lead the group through a series of seated stretches, gentle movements, and mindfulness practices, encouraging participants to move with awareness and intention. Chair yoga circles provide a supportive space for caregivers to come together, share experiences, and rejuvenate body and mind.

Chair Yoga Games: Infuse your chair yoga sessions with fun and playfulness by incorporating chair yoga games. Explore simple games such as "Chair Yoga Simon Says" or "Chair Yoga Musical Chairs," where participants perform various chair yoga poses in response to verbal cues or music. Games add an element of joy and laughter to your chair yoga practice, fostering a sense of camaraderie and light-heartedness among participants.

Group Meditation and Relaxation: Dedicate time at the end of your chair yoga session for a group meditation or relaxation practice. Guide participants through a guided imagery meditation, inviting them to visualize a peaceful scene or positive affirmation. Alternatively, lead a progressive muscle relaxation exercise, encouraging participants to release tension from head to toe. Group meditation and relaxation foster a sense of unity and collective calm, promoting emotional well-being and stress relief.

Chair Yoga Workshops and Retreats: Organize or attend chair yoga workshops or retreats designed specifically for caregivers or community groups. These immersive experiences offer an opportunity to deepen your chair yoga practice, learn new techniques, and connect with like-minded individuals in a supportive environment. Chair yoga workshops and retreats provide a valuable opportunity for caregivers to recharge, rejuvenate, and cultivate a sense of belonging within a supportive community.

Caregiving can foster a sense of community and connection while advancing their physical, mental, and social well-being by experimenting with partner and group chair yoga sessions. Chair yoga is a potent method to create important connections and a feeling of community among carers, whether you practise with a spouse, in a group, or at a workshop or retreat.

Building Support Networks and Seeking Assistance

Caregiving can often feel like a solitary journey, but it's essential to remember that you don't have to navigate it alone. Building support networks and seeking assistance are crucial steps in maintaining your well-being as a caregiver. Here are some strategies to help you cultivate a strong support system and access the help you need:

Reach Out to Family and Friends: Don't hesitate to lean on your family and friends for support. Share your caregiving responsibilities with trusted loved ones and communicate openly about your needs and challenges. Whether it's providing respite care, running errands, or simply lending a listening ear, involving family and friends can lighten your load and strengthen your connections.

Join Caregiver Support Groups: Seek out caregiver support groups in your community or online where you can connect with others who are going through similar experiences. These groups offer a safe space to share your feelings, exchange practical tips, and receive emotional support from individuals who understand firsthand the demands of caregiving. Participating in support groups can alleviate feelings of isolation and provide valuable resources and guidance

Attend Educational Workshops and Events: Look for educational workshops, seminars, and events focused on caregiving-related topics. These gatherings not only offer valuable information and resources but also provide opportunities to connect with professionals, experts, and fellow caregivers. Attend lectures, panel discussions, and Q&A sessions to gain insights into caregiving best practices, self-care techniques, and available support services.

Explore Community Resources: Take advantage of community resources and services designed to support caregivers. Contact local senior centers, hospitals, and social service agencies to inquire about caregiver support programs, respite care services, and educational workshops. Many communities offer free or low-cost resources such as support groups, counseling services, and caregiver training programs to help caregivers cope with their responsibilities effectively.

Seek Professional Help: Don't hesitate to seek professional assistance when needed. Reach out to healthcare providers, therapists, or counselors who specialize in caregiver support and mental health. Professional guidance can help you navigate complex emotions, manage caregiver stress, and develop coping strategies tailored to your unique situation. Consider individual therapy, counseling sessions, or caregiver coaching to address your specific needs and challenges.

Utilize Technology and Online Resources: Explore digital tools, mobile apps, and online platforms designed to support caregivers. From virtual support groups and telehealth services to caregiver forums and educational webinars, technology offers a wealth of resources at your fingertips. Take advantage of online communities, social media groups, and caregiver websites to connect with peers, access information, and find inspiration on your caregiving journey.

Delegate Tasks and Responsibilities: Recognize that you can't do it all and don't hesitate to delegate tasks and responsibilities when necessary. Whether it's hiring professional caregivers, utilizing home care services, or enlisting the help of volunteers, outsourcing certain tasks can provide much-needed relief and allow you to focus on your own well-being. Prioritize self-care and set boundaries to prevent burnout and exhaustion.

Building support networks and seeking assistance are essential components of effective caregiving. By reaching out to family and friends, joining support groups, accessing community resources, seeking professional help, utilizing technology, and delegating tasks, caregivers can create a robust support system to help them navigate the challenges of caregiving with greater ease and resilience.

The Power of Sharing Experiences and Resources

In the journey of caregiving, the power of sharing experiences and resources cannot be overstated. Caregivers often find solace, support, and valuable insights by connecting with others who understand their challenges and triumphs. Here's why sharing experiences and resources can be transformative for caregivers:

Validation and Understanding: When caregivers connect with others who share similar experiences, they find validation and understanding. Sharing stories, challenges, and triumphs with fellow caregivers helps normalize their experiences and feelings. Knowing that they are not alone in their struggles can alleviate feelings of isolation and offer much-needed emotional support.

Practical Tips and Advice: Caregivers learn valuable tips, strategies, and practical advice from others who have walked a similar path. Whether it's learning how to manage caregiver stress, navigate complex healthcare systems, or cope with difficult emotions, sharing resources and insights can provide caregivers with actionable guidance and solutions to common challenges.

Empowerment and Resilience: Connecting with a supportive community empowers caregivers to face their responsibilities with resilience and determination. By sharing stories of resilience, perseverance, and self-care, caregivers inspire and uplift one another. They gain strength from knowing that others have faced similar obstacles and overcome them, fostering a sense of solidarity and hope.

Access to Resources and Support: Sharing experiences and resources opens doors to a wealth of support networks, services, and resources. Caregivers exchange information about helpful books, websites, support groups, and community services that can enhance their caregiving journey. By tapping into these resources, caregivers access a broader range of support and assistance tailored to their needs.

Emotional Connection and Camaraderie: Building connections with other caregivers fosters a sense of camaraderie and emotional connection. Caregivers find comfort and companionship in sharing their joys and sorrows with others who understand the unique challenges of caregiving. These connections provide a safe space for caregivers to express themselves authentically and receive unconditional support.

Reduced Stress and Burnout: Engaging with a supportive community reduces caregiver stress and prevents burnout. By sharing their experiences and challenges, caregivers alleviate feelings of burden and overwhelm. They gain perspective, insights, and coping strategies that help them manage stress more effectively and maintain their well-being.

Advocacy and Awareness: Caregivers who share their experiences become powerful advocates for themselves and others. By raising awareness about the realities of caregiving, they amplify their voices and advocate for policy changes, improved support services, and greater recognition of caregiver needs. Sharing stories of caregiving challenges and triumphs helps educate the public and policymakers about the importance of supporting caregivers.

In conclusion, the power of sharing experiences and resources lies in its ability to validate, empower, and support caregivers on their journey. By connecting with others, caregivers gain practical tips, emotional support, and access to valuable resources that enhance their well-being and resilience. Together, caregivers create a community of strength, compassion, and solidarity, transforming the caregiving experience into one of shared purpose and connection.

CHAPTER 9
Kundalini Yoga Practices for Caregivers

Introduction to Kundalini Yoga and Its Benefits for Caregivers

Kundalini Yoga, often referred to as the "yoga of awareness," is a powerful practice that integrates physical postures, breathwork, meditation, and mantra chanting to awaken the dormant energy within the body and promote holistic well-being. Rooted in ancient yogic traditions, Kundalini Yoga offers a unique approach to self-discovery, healing, and spiritual growth. Here's an introduction to Kundalini Yoga and how its benefits are particularly relevant for caregivers:

1. Awakening Vital Energy: At the core of Kundalini Yoga is the awakening of Kundalini energy, often depicted as a coiled serpent at the base of the spine. Through specific yoga techniques, practitioners awaken this dormant energy and allow it to rise through the chakras, or energy centers, along the spine. This process of awakening vital energy helps caregivers replenish their energy reserves, combat fatigue, and restore balance to the mind, body, and spirit.

2. Stress Reduction and Relaxation: Kundalini Yoga offers powerful tools for stress reduction and relaxation. The practice includes dynamic movements, breathwork, and meditation techniques designed to release tension from the body and calm the mind. Caregivers can use Kundalini Yoga practices to alleviate stress, anxiety, and overwhelm, allowing them to experience deep relaxation and inner peace amidst their caregiving responsibilities.

3. Emotional Healing and Balance: Kundalini Yoga facilitates emotional healing and balance by working with the body's energy system and clearing emotional blockages. Through specific yoga postures, breathwork, and meditation practices, caregivers can release stored emotions, such as grief, anger, and resentment, and cultivate a greater sense of emotional equilibrium. Kundalini Yoga empowers caregivers to navigate their emotions with grace and compassion, fostering emotional resilience and well-being.

4. Cultivating Mindfulness and Presence: Kundalini Yoga emphasizes the cultivation of mindfulness and presence in every moment. Caregivers learn to anchor themselves in the present moment through focused attention, conscious breathing, and mindful movement. This practice of mindfulness allows caregivers to approach their caregiving duties with greater awareness, clarity, and presence, enhancing the quality of their interactions and fostering deeper connections with their loved ones.

5. Enhancing Intuition and Self-awareness: Kundalini Yoga practices promote the development of intuition and self-awareness, enabling caregivers to tap into their inner wisdom and guidance. Through meditation, visualization, and mantra chanting, caregivers can access deeper layers of consciousness and intuition, gaining insights into their own needs, desires, and limitations. This heightened self-awareness empowers caregivers to make informed decisions, set healthy boundaries, and prioritize self-care effectively.

6. Strengthening Resilience and Adaptability: Kundalini Yoga builds resilience and adaptability by cultivating a sense of inner strength and flexibility. Caregivers develop physical, mental, and emotional resilience through the challenges of Kundalini Yoga practices, such as holding challenging postures and navigating intense breathwork. This resilience translates into greater adaptability and resourcefulness in the face of adversity, enabling caregivers to navigate the ups and downs of their caregiving journey with grace and fortitude.

7. Nourishing Spiritual Connection: Kundalini Yoga nourishes caregivers' spiritual connection and fosters a sense of interconnectedness with the universe. Through meditation, mantra chanting, and devotion, caregivers deepen their connection to their inner divine essence and the greater cosmos. This spiritual connection provides solace, inspiration, and guidance, anchoring caregivers in a sense of purpose and meaning amidst the complexities of caregiving.

In summary, Kundalini Yoga offers caregivers a holistic approach to self-care and well-being, addressing their physical, emotional, mental, and spiritual needs. By incorporating Kundalini Yoga practices into their daily routine, caregivers can awaken their vital energy, reduce stress, cultivate emotional balance, enhance mindfulness, strengthen resilience, and nourish their spiritual connection. Through the transformative power of Kundalini Yoga, caregivers embark on a journey of self-discovery, healing, and empowerment, reclaiming their inner radiance and vitality amidst the demands of caregiving.

Key Kundalini Yoga Practices for Stress Relief and Self-care

Kundalini Yoga offers a rich array of practices specifically tailored to help caregivers manage stress, cultivate self-care, and restore balance in their lives. These key practices encompass a variety of techniques, including dynamic movements, breathwork, meditation, and mantra chanting, all aimed at promoting holistic well-being. Here are some essential Kundalini Yoga practices for caregivers:

1. Breath of Fire (Agni Pran): This rapid, rhythmic breathwork technique is a cornerstone of Kundalini Yoga, known for its energizing and purifying effects. By rapidly inhaling and exhaling through the nose, caregivers activate the body's vital energy, oxygenate the blood, and release toxins from the system. Breath of Fire is particularly effective for boosting energy levels, enhancing mental clarity, and reducing stress and anxiety.

2. Cat-Cow Stretch (Marjaryasana-Bitilasana): This gentle spinal movement sequence helps caregivers release tension from the spine, improve flexibility, and promote relaxation. By alternating between arching and rounding the back while synchronizing movement with breath, caregivers massage the spine, stimulate the nervous system, and create a sense of fluidity and ease in the body.

3. Sat Nam Meditation: Sat Nam, meaning "truth is my identity," is a powerful mantra used in Kundalini Yoga to connect with one's true essence and cultivate inner peace. Caregivers can practice Sat Nam meditation by silently repeating the mantra while sitting in a comfortable position, focusing on the breath, and allowing the vibration of the mantra to resonate within the body and mind. This meditation promotes self-awareness, clarity, and emotional balance.

4. Heart Center Activation (Anahata Chakra): Kundalini Yoga offers specific practices to activate and balance the heart chakra, the center of love, compassion, and emotional well-being. Caregivers can practice heart-opening postures, such as Camel Pose (Ustrasana) and Cobra Pose (Bhujangasana), to open the chest, expand the heart center, and release emotional blockages. These practices cultivate a sense of compassion, empathy, and connection with oneself and others.

5. Relaxing Nervous System (Shavasana): Shavasana, or Corpse Pose, is a deeply relaxing posture that allows caregivers to release physical and mental tension, rejuvenate the body, and calm the nervous system. By lying flat on their backs with arms and legs comfortably spread, caregivers can practice conscious relaxation, surrendering to the support of the earth and allowing tension to melt away. Shavasana promotes deep rest, stress relief, and a profound sense of inner peace.

6. Grounding Earth Meditation: This meditation practice helps caregivers cultivate a sense of grounding, stability, and security amidst the demands of caregiving. By visualizing themselves rooted to the earth like a sturdy tree, caregivers connect with the grounding energy of the earth, anchoring themselves in the present moment and finding stability amidst life's challenges. This meditation fosters resilience, inner strength, and a sense of rootedness in times of stress.

7. Self-Compassion and Forgiveness: Kundalini Yoga encourages caregivers to practice self-compassion and forgiveness as essential components of self-care. Through meditation, reflection, and mantra chanting, caregivers can cultivate love and acceptance towards themselves, embracing their imperfections and honoring their journey. By letting go of self-criticism and judgment, caregivers create space for healing, self-love, and emotional well-being.

By adding four essential Kundalini Yoga exercises into their daily routine, carers can better manage stress, practise self-care, and improve their general well-being. In the middle of the responsibilities of caregiving, carers regain their inner balance, strength, and vigour by setting aside time to attend to their physical, emotional, and spiritual needs through Kundalini Yoga.

Deep Listening Meditation

Deep Listening Meditation is a profound practice that invites caregivers to cultivate inner stillness, heightened awareness, and deep connection with themselves and their surroundings. In the midst of caregiving responsibilities and life's demands, this meditation offers a sanctuary of peace and presence, allowing caregivers to replenish their energy, find clarity, and access inner guidance.

To practice Deep Listening Meditation

Find a Quiet Space: Choose a quiet and comfortable space where you can sit undisturbed for the duration of the meditation. Ensure that you are seated in a relaxed posture, with your spine comfortably aligned and your hands resting gently on your lap.

Settle into Stillness: Close your eyes softly and take a few deep breaths to settle into the present moment. Allow your body to relax and release any tension or tightness you may be holding. Feel the support of the earth beneath you, grounding and anchoring you in the present moment.

Cultivate Inner Silence: Shift your awareness inward and begin to cultivate inner silence by letting go of mental chatter and distractions. Allow your thoughts to gently dissolve, like clouds drifting across the sky, as you enter a state of deep relaxation and receptivity.

Deepen Your Listening: As you settle into stillness, shift your focus to the act of listening—listening not only with your ears but with your entire being. Tune into the subtle sounds around you, whether it's the rustling of leaves, the chirping of birds, or the gentle rhythm of your breath.

Open Your Heart: As you deepen your listening, open your heart to receive whatever arises in your awareness. Allow yourself to be fully present with whatever thoughts, emotions, or sensations may arise, without judgment or resistance. Embrace each moment with an attitude of openness, curiosity, and compassion.

Connect with Your Inner Wisdom: As you continue to listen deeply, you may find that insights, intuitions, or inner guidance begins to emerge. Trust in the wisdom of your inner voice and allow it to guide you on your journey. Stay receptive and open to whatever messages or revelations may arise.

Rest in Stillness: After a period of deep listening, gently release your focus and allow yourself to rest in stillness for a few moments. Bask in the sense of peace, clarity, and inner knowing that arises from this practice, knowing that you can return to it whenever you need to find centering and solace.

Deep Listening Meditation offers caregivers a powerful tool for cultivating presence, inner peace, and self-awareness amidst the busyness of their lives. By dedicating time to listen deeply to themselves and their surroundings, caregivers nourish their spirits, replenish their energy, and deepen their connection with the present moment.

Kriya for Hard Decisions

Caregiving often involves making difficult decisions that can weigh heavily on the mind and heart. The Kriya for Hard Decisions is a Kundalini Yoga practice designed to provide caregivers with clarity, courage, and inner strength when faced with challenging choices.

To practice the Kriya for Hard Decisions:

Prepare Your Space: Find a quiet and peaceful space where you can practice without distractions. Sit comfortably on a chair or cushion with your spine straight and your hands resting on your knees.

Begin with Tuning In: Close your eyes and take a few deep breaths to center yourself. Then, bring your hands together in prayer position at the center of your chest. Inhale deeply, and as you exhale, chant the mantra "Ong Namo Guru Dev Namo" three times. This mantra helps to connect you with your inner wisdom and the wisdom of the universe.

Kriya Sequence: The Kriya for Hard Decisions consists of a series of specific movements, breathwork, and meditation techniques. Follow the instructions carefully and perform each component with focused awareness and intention.

Stretch and Warm-Up: Begin by gently stretching your arms overhead and then twisting gently from side to side to release tension in the spine.

Breath of Fire: Sit with a straight spine and place your hands on your knees. Begin rapid and rhythmic breathing through your nose, pumping your navel point in and out with each breath. Continue for 1-3 minutes, focusing on the sensation of energy moving through your body.

Meditation: Sit quietly with your eyes closed and bring your attention to the area just above your eyebrows, known as the third eye center. Visualize a clear, bright light shining from this point, illuminating your mind and providing clarity. Hold this visualization for 3-11 minutes, allowing yourself to feel grounded and centered.

Closing: To conclude the practice, inhale deeply and raise your arms overhead, stretching upward with your fingertips. Exhale as you lower your arms back down to your sides. Take a moment to express gratitude for the clarity and insight you've received during the practice.

Reflect and Integrate: After completing the Kriya, take some time to reflect on any insights or guidance that arose during the practice. Trust in your inner wisdom and know that you have the strength and courage to make the decisions that are best for you and your loved ones.

The Kriya for Hard Decisions is a powerful tool for caregivers to access their inner guidance and find clarity in times of uncertainty. By practicing this kriya regularly, caregivers can cultivate resilience, trust in themselves, and the confidence to navigate even the most challenging situations with grace and wisdom.

Techniques for Coping with Loss and Grief

Caring for a loved one can bring immense joy and fulfillment, but it can also come with its share of loss and grief. Whether it's the loss of independence, the decline in health, or the eventual passing of a loved one, caregivers often face profound feelings of sorrow and mourning. Kundalini Yoga offers powerful techniques to help caregivers navigate through the journey of loss and grief with strength, compassion, and resilience.

Here are some Kundalini Yoga techniques for coping with loss and grief:

Breathwork for Emotional Release: Kundalini Yoga incorporates various breathing techniques, known as pranayama, to help release pent-up emotions and promote emotional healing. One such technique is the Breath of Fire, a rapid and rhythmic breath that helps to energize the body and clear the mind. Practice Breath of Fire for 3-5 minutes, focusing on releasing any sadness or grief with each exhalation.

Meditation for Healing: Meditation is a powerful tool for processing emotions and finding inner peace amidst the storm of grief. One effective meditation practice is the Healing Meditation for Grief, which involves sitting in a comfortable position and silently chanting the mantra **"Ra Ma Da Sa"** while visualizing healing energy flowing through your body and soothing your heart. Practice this meditation for *11-31 minutes daily* to experience profound healing and emotional relief.

Heart-Opening Yoga Poses: Certain yoga poses can help to open the heart center and release stored emotions. Practice gentle backbends such as Cobra Pose (Bhujangasana) or Bridge Pose (Setu Bandhasana) to stretch and strengthen the muscles of the chest and upper back, allowing for a release of emotional tension and grief.

Journaling and Self-Reflection: Writing can be a therapeutic way to process emotions and gain clarity during times of grief. Set aside time each day to journal about your feelings, thoughts, and experiences related to caregiving and loss. Allow yourself to express your emotions freely on paper, without judgment or inhibition.

Seeking Support and Community: Remember that you're not alone in your journey of grief. Reach out to friends, family members, or support groups for comfort, understanding, and companionship. Connecting with others who are going through similar experiences can provide validation, empathy, and solace.

Honoring Rituals and Remembrance: Create meaningful rituals or ceremonies to honor the memory of your loved one and acknowledge the significance of your caregiving journey. Light a candle, say a prayer, or create a memorial altar with photos and mementos that evoke feelings of love, gratitude, and connection.

By incorporating these Kundalini Yoga techniques into your daily routine, you can cultivate resilience, find solace amidst grief, and honor the sacred journey of caregiving with compassion and grace. Allow yourself the space to grieve, heal, and ultimately, find peace amidst the challenges and joys of caregiving.

CHAPTER 10
Maintaining Balance and Resilience

Cultivating Self-esteem and Awareness

Caregiving often entails putting the needs of others before your own, which can sometimes lead to feelings of self-doubt, inadequacy, or low self-esteem. Cultivating self-esteem and awareness is essential for caregivers to maintain a sense of confidence, self-worth, and resilience amidst the challenges they face. Kundalini Yoga offers powerful practices to help caregivers cultivate self-esteem and awareness, allowing them to approach their caregiving role with greater clarity, compassion, and strength.

Here are some Kundalini Yoga techniques for cultivating self-esteem and awareness:

Mirror Meditation: Sit comfortably in front of a mirror and gaze into your own eyes. Take several deep breaths to center yourself, and then repeat affirmations such as "I am worthy," "I am capable," and "I am enough" while maintaining eye contact with yourself. Allow yourself to receive these positive affirmations deeply into your being, nurturing a sense of self-love, acceptance, and worthiness.

Kriya for Self-empowerment: Practice Kundalini Yoga kriyas (sets of exercises) specifically designed to boost self-confidence and empowerment. One such kriya is the Ego Eradicator, which involves sitting in a comfortable cross-legged position, raising the arms overhead in a V-shape, and practicing Breath of Fire for 1-3 minutes. This powerful kriya helps to clear self-limiting beliefs and energize the body, allowing you to step into your power with confidence and clarity.

Body Scan Meditation: Practice a guided body scan meditation to increase self-awareness and presence in the moment. Lie down in a comfortable position and close your eyes. Begin by bringing your attention to your breath, and then slowly scan through each part of your body, from head to toe, noticing any sensations, tensions, or areas of discomfort. Simply observe without judgment or resistance, allowing yourself to fully inhabit your body and experience the present moment with awareness and acceptance.

Journaling and Reflective Writing: Set aside time each day for reflective writing and self-inquiry. Use journal prompts such as "What do I appreciate about myself?" "What are my strengths as a caregiver?" and "What can I do to nourish myself today?" to explore your thoughts, feelings, and inner wisdom. Writing can be a powerful tool for self-discovery, allowing you to uncover hidden beliefs, patterns, and strengths that support your sense of self-esteem and awareness.

Mindful Movement Practices: Engage in mindful movement practices such as walking meditation, gentle yoga, or tai chi to cultivate present-moment awareness and embodiment. Pay attention to the sensations of movement in your body, the rhythm of your breath, and the subtle shifts in energy as you move mindfully through space. These practices help to ground you in the present moment and foster a deeper connection to yourself and your inner resources.

You can cultivate a sense of self-worth, self-awareness, and self-compassion that helps you in your job as a caregiver by implementing these Kundalini Yoga practices into your everyday practice. Remind yourself that you deserve respect, love, and attention from others as well as from yourself. Give yourself permission to accept your innate merit and confidently and gracefully assume your role as a caregiver.

Practices for Self-expression and Purpose

As a caregiver, it's easy to lose sight of your own needs and desires amidst the demands of caregiving. However, nurturing your sense of self-expression and purpose is essential for maintaining balance and resilience in your caregiving journey. Kundalini Yoga offers powerful practices to help you reconnect with your inner passions, creativity, and sense of purpose, allowing you to express yourself authentically and live with greater fulfillment and joy.

Here are some Kundalini Yoga practices for self-expression and purpose:

Creative Visualization: Take time each day to visualize your ideal life, focusing on your passions, goals, and aspirations. Sit comfortably in a quiet space, close your eyes, and imagine yourself living a life filled with purpose, joy, and fulfillment. Visualize yourself engaging in activities that bring you happiness and fulfillment, and allow yourself to feel the emotions associated with living your best life. Creative visualization helps to align your thoughts, beliefs, and actions with your deepest desires, empowering you to manifest your dreams and live with greater purpose.

Soul Gazing Meditation: Practice soul gazing meditation with a trusted partner or loved one to deepen your connection and cultivate a sense of shared purpose and intimacy. Sit facing each other in a comfortable position, maintaining eye contact, and allowing yourselves to gaze into each other's eyes without speaking. This practice helps to create a profound sense of connection and understanding, fostering empathy, compassion, and mutual support in your caregiving relationship.

Journaling and Creative Writing: Set aside time each day for journaling and creative writing to express your thoughts, feelings, and innermost desires. Use writing prompts such as "What brings me joy?" "What am I passionate about?" and "What is my purpose in life?" to explore your inner landscape and uncover the truths that resonate deeply with your soul. Writing can be a powerful tool for self-expression and self-discovery, allowing you to tap into your creativity and intuition and connect with your authentic self.

Dance and Movement Practices: Explore the expressive power of dance and movement to release pent-up emotions, awaken your creativity, and connect with your body's wisdom. Put on your favorite music and allow yourself to move freely and spontaneously, expressing yourself through dance and movement. Pay attention to the sensations, emotions, and energy flowing through your body, allowing yourself to move in ways that feel natural and authentic. Dance and movement practices help to liberate your creative energy, ignite your passion, and cultivate a deeper sense of purpose and aliveness.

Service and Contribution: Find ways to serve others and contribute to causes that are meaningful to you, whether through volunteering, acts of kindness, or sharing your skills and talents with others. Serving others not only brings joy and fulfillment but also connects you with a sense of purpose and meaning beyond yourself. Look for opportunities to make a positive impact in your community and the world, and allow yourself to experience the deep satisfaction that comes from making a difference in the lives of others. You can cultivate your sense of self-expression and purpose by implementing these Kundalini Yoga practices into your daily routine. This will enable you to live a life that is more joyful, fulfilling, and meaningful while providing care for others. Never forget that you deserve to have a life that is in line with your greatest aspirations and passions and to express yourself honestly. Give yourself permission to accept your special abilities and gifts, and shine brightly for the benefit of both yourself and other people.

Finding Belonging and Connection Through Yoga

As a caregiver, it's common to feel isolated and disconnected from others due to the demands of caregiving. However, practicing yoga can offer you a sense of belonging and connection to a supportive community, both on and off the mat. Yoga provides a safe and inclusive space where you can connect with like-minded individuals, share your experiences, and receive support and encouragement from others who understand your challenges.

Here are some ways to find belonging and connection through yoga:

Join a Yoga Class: Explore local yoga studios or community centers to find classes specifically tailored for caregivers or individuals experiencing similar life challenges. Joining a yoga class provides an opportunity to connect with others who share your experiences, forming bonds of friendship and support that extend beyond the yoga mat. Look for classes that focus on gentle, restorative yoga or chair yoga, allowing you to practice in a safe and accessible environment.

Attend Yoga Workshops and Retreats: Consider attending yoga workshops or retreats designed for caregivers, offering a deeper exploration of yoga practices and self-care techniques in a supportive and nurturing setting. These events provide an opportunity to connect with a community of caregivers, share stories and insights, and learn from experienced yoga teachers and wellness professionals. Retreats offer a chance to immerse yourself in the practice of yoga, relaxation, and self-reflection, fostering deep connections and lasting friendships with fellow participants.

Online Yoga Communities: Explore online yoga communities and forums dedicated to caregivers, where you can connect with others virtually and share your experiences, challenges, and triumphs. Online communities provide a supportive space for caregivers to seek advice, offer encouragement, and find inspiration from others on similar journeys. Participate in virtual yoga classes, workshops, and discussions, allowing you to connect with a global community of caregivers and yoga practitioners from the comfort of your own home.

Create a Yoga Circle: Form a small group of caregivers in your local community who are interested in practicing yoga together regularly. Meet in person or virtually to practice yoga, share resources, and offer mutual support and encouragement. Creating a yoga circle allows you to build meaningful connections with others who understand and empathize with your caregiving experiences, fostering a sense of belonging and camaraderie.

Yoga Outreach Programs: Explore yoga outreach programs and initiatives that offer yoga classes and mindfulness practices to underserved populations, including caregivers, seniors, and individuals facing health challenges. Volunteer with local organizations or nonprofits that provide yoga classes in hospitals, nursing homes, and community centers, offering your time and expertise to support others on their healing journeys. Engaging in yoga outreach allows you to give back to your community while connecting with individuals from diverse backgrounds and experiences. By finding belonging and connection through yoga, you can cultivate a supportive community of fellow caregivers and yoga practitioners who understand and support you on your caregiving journey. Whether you join a yoga class, attend workshops and retreats, participate in online communities, or create a yoga circle, know that you are not alone and that there is a community of like-minded individuals waiting to welcome you with open arms. Embrace the opportunity to connect, share, and grow together through the transformative power of yoga.

CHAPTER 11
Integrating Chair Yoga and Kundalini Yoga

Creating a Holistic Self-care Routine

Integrating chair yoga and Kundalini yoga into your daily routine can significantly enhance your overall well-being and resilience as a caregiver. By incorporating these practices into your self-care routine, you can nurture your physical, mental, and emotional health, allowing you to navigate the challenges of caregiving with greater ease and grace. Here's how to create a holistic self-care routine that combines chair yoga and Kundalini yoga practices:

Morning Chair Yoga Practice: Start your day with a gentle chair yoga practice to awaken your body and mind, preparing yourself for the day ahead. Begin with deep breathing exercises to center yourself and clear your mind. Then, move through a series of gentle stretches and movements to release tension and stiffness in your muscles and joints. Focus on poses that promote flexibility, strength, and balance, such as seated twists, side stretches, and forward folds. Allow yourself to move with awareness and mindfulness, tuning into the sensations in your body and breath.

Kundalini Yoga Kriya: Incorporate a Kundalini yoga Kriya into your morning routine to energize your body, uplift your spirit, and enhance your mental clarity. Choose a Kriya that resonates with your current needs and intentions, whether it's for stress relief, emotional balance, or inner strength. Practice dynamic movements, breathwork, and meditation techniques to awaken your Kundalini energy and align your chakras. Allow yourself to fully engage with the practice, surrendering to the transformative power of Kundalini yoga to uplift and inspire you.

Midday Mindfulness Break: Take a midday mindfulness break to pause, reset, and recharge amidst the busyness of caregiving. Find a quiet space where you can sit comfortably and practice mindfulness meditation or deep relaxation techniques. Close your eyes and focus on your breath, allowing yourself to become fully present in the moment. Release any tension or stress held in your body and mind, cultivating a sense of inner peace and tranquility. Use this time to reconnect with yourself and nourish your soul, setting aside worries and distractions as you rest in the stillness of the present moment.

Evening Chair Yoga Practice: Wind down your day with a soothing chair yoga practice to relax your body and prepare for restful sleep. Practice gentle stretches and restorative poses to release physical tension and promote deep relaxation. Focus on poses that target areas of the body prone to stress and tension, such as the neck, shoulders, and lower back. Incorporate mindful breathing techniques and guided relaxation exercises to quiet your mind and soothe your nervous system. Allow yourself to surrender to the healing power of yoga, letting go of the day's worries and embracing a sense of peace and serenity.

Bedtime Kundalini Meditation: End your day with a calming Kundalini meditation practice to promote restful sleep and inner tranquility. Choose a meditation technique that promotes relaxation, such as chanting a soothing mantra or practicing yoga

Nidra. Settle into a comfortable position, close your eyes, and allow yourself to let go of any remaining tension or stress. Surrender to the gentle rhythm of your breath and the peacefulness of the present moment, inviting a sense of deep relaxation and inner stillness. Allow the healing energy of Kundalini meditation to envelop you, guiding you into a restful and rejuvenating night's sleep.

By creating a holistic self-care routine that incorporates chair yoga and Kundalini yoga practices, you can nurture your physical, mental, and emotional well-being as a caregiver. Make self-care a priority in your daily life, honoring your body, mind, and spirit with the restorative power of yoga. Embrace these practices as sacred rituals of self-love and self-care, allowing them to support you in your journey of caregiving and self-discovery.

Combining Chair Yoga and Kundalini Yoga Practices for Maximum Benefits

Integrating chair yoga and Kundalini yoga into your self-care routine offers a powerful synergy that enhances your overall well-being and resilience as a caregiver. By combining these two modalities, you can access a comprehensive toolkit of practices to support your physical, mental, and emotional health, enabling you to navigate the demands of caregiving with greater ease and grace. Here's how to effectively combine chair yoga and Kundalini yoga practices for maximum benefits:

Chair Yoga Warm-up: Begin your practice with a gentle chair yoga warm-up to prepare your body for deeper exploration and movement. Focus on gentle stretches and mobility exercises that target key areas of tension and stiffness, such as the neck, shoulders, and hips. Incorporate mindful breathing techniques to center yourself and cultivate a sense of inner calm and presence. Use this time to connect with your body and breath, tuning in to any sensations or areas of discomfort.

Kundalini Yoga Kriyas: After warming up, transition into Kundalini yoga kriyas, which are dynamic, repetitive movements combined with breathwork and meditation. Choose kriyas that address specific areas of concern or focus, such as reducing stress, increasing energy, or promoting mental clarity. Examples include spinal twists, arm swings, and leg lifts performed while seated in a chair. Focus on moving with intention and awareness, allowing the energy to flow freely throughout your body.

Breathwork and Meditation: Incorporate pranayama (breathwork) and meditation techniques from both chair yoga and Kundalini yoga traditions to calm the mind, balance the nervous system, and enhance emotional well-being. Practice deep belly breathing, alternate nostril breathing, or Breath of Fire to regulate your breath and quiet the chatter of the mind. Explore meditation practices such as mindfulness meditation, mantra meditation, or guided visualization to cultivate inner peace and clarity.

Integration and Reflection: Take time at the end of your practice to integrate the physical, mental, and emotional benefits of your yoga practice. Sit quietly for a few moments, allowing yourself to bask in the afterglow of your practice and to reflect on any insights or revelations that may have arisen. Express gratitude for the opportunity to nurture yourself and acknowledge the resilience and strength that resides within you.

By combining chair yoga and Kundalini yoga practices in your self-care routine, you can cultivate a deeper sense of well-being, resilience, and balance as a caregiver. Experiment with different practices and techniques to discover what works best for you, and remember to honor your body's needs and limitations as you embark on this transformative journey of self-discovery and healing.

CONCLUSION
Celebrating Your Self-care Journey

Committing to Continued Self-care Practices

As you reach the conclusion of this transformative journey, it's essential to acknowledge the progress you've made and commit to ongoing self-care practices that nurture your well-being as a caregiver. While this journey may have been filled with challenges and obstacles, it's also been marked by moments of growth, resilience, and self-discovery. By committing to continued self-care practices, you honor the investment you've made in your health and well-being, ensuring that you can continue to show up fully for yourself and those you care for.

Reflect on Your Progress: Take a moment to reflect on how far you've come since beginning this journey. Celebrate the small victories and milestones you've achieved along the way, whether it's cultivating a daily yoga practice, prioritizing restorative sleep, or setting healthy boundaries in your caregiving role. Acknowledge the inner strength and resilience you've developed as you've navigated the ups and downs of caregiving.

Identify Your Self-care Priorities: Consider what self-care practices have been most effective and beneficial for you during this journey. Whether it's chair yoga, Kundalini yoga, mindfulness meditation, or simply carving out time for yourself each day, identify the self-care activities that bring you the greatest sense of peace, balance, and rejuvenation. These practices will serve as the foundation of your ongoing self-care routine.

Create a Sustainable Self-care Plan: Develop a sustainable self-care plan that incorporates your preferred practices and aligns with your lifestyle and schedule. Set realistic goals and intentions for your self-care journey, making sure to prioritize consistency and commitment. Consider enlisting the support of loved ones, healthcare professionals, or support groups to help you stay accountable and motivated along the way.

Practice Self-compassion: Be gentle with yourself as you navigate the ups and downs of your self-care journey. Recognize that self-care is not a linear process and that there will be days when you may struggle to prioritize your well-being. Instead of judging yourself harshly, practice self-compassion and kindness, offering yourself the same love and care that you extend to others.

Celebrate Your Successes: Celebrate your successes and achievements along the way, no matter how small they may seem. Whether it's taking a few moments to savor a peaceful yoga practice, enjoying a leisurely walk in nature, or simply pausing to breathe deeply and connect with the present moment, each act of self-care is a victory worth celebrating.

By committing to continued self-care practices, you honor yourself as a caregiver and recognize the importance of nurturing your own well-being. Embrace this journey with an open heart and a sense of curiosity, knowing that each step you take towards self-care brings you closer to a life of balance, resilience, and fulfilment. As you move forward, may you find strength in your self-care practices and experience the profound benefits they offer, both on and off the mat.

Thank you for choosing **Chair Yoga for Caregivers**: Self-care Practices to Relieve Stress and Restore Balance as your guide. We've included an online video instruction to improve your experience and help you better grasp the chair yoga techniques that are described in this book.

Simply scan the **QR code** provided below using your smartphone or tablet camera to access the video tutorial. This tutorial will guide you through each exercise step-by-step, ensuring proper form and alignment as you practice.

We encourage you to utilize this valuable resource to maximize the benefits of your chair yoga practice and support your overall well-being. Remember, consistency is key, so carve out a few moments each day to dedicate to your self-care practice.

Thank you for investing in your health and well-being. We wish you joy, peace, and rejuvenation on your self-care journey.

www.ingramcontent.com/pod-product-compliance
Lightning Source LLC
Chambersburg PA
CBHW061642250726

48659CB00004B/1349